Psychiatry and Religion

Grant Miller

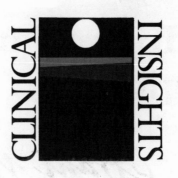
CLINICAL INSIGHTS

Psychiatry and Religion: Overlapping Concerns

Edited by
LILLIAN H. ROBINSON, M.D.

Professor of Psychiatry and Pediatrics; and Training and Supervising Analyst, Analytic Medicine Program, Department of Psychiatry and Neurology, Tulane University School of Medicine, New Orleans

AMERICAN PSYCHIATRIC PRESS, INC.
Washington, D.C.

© 1986 American Psychiatric Press, Inc.

Manufactured in the U.S.A.

The paper used in this publication meets the minimum requirements of American National Standard for Information Sciences—Permanence of Papers for Printed Library Materials, ANSI Z39.48-1984. ∞^{TM}

Library of Congress Cataloging in Publication Data

Main entry under title:

Psychiatry and religion.

(Clinical insights)
Grew out of a symposium presented at the 138th Annual Meeting of the American Psychiatric Association, a joint session of the Association and the American Academy of Psychoanalysis.
Includes bibliographies.
1. Psychiatry and religion—Congresses. 2.—Psychoanalysis and religion —Congresses. 3. Pastoral psychology—Congresses. I. Robinson, Lillian H., 1918- . II. American Psychiatric Association. Meeting (138th : 1985 : Dallas, Tex.) III. American Academy of Psychoanalysis. IV. Series. [DNLM: 1. Pastoral care— Congresses. 2. Psychiatry—Congresses. 3. Religion and Medicine—Congresses. WM 61 P974 1985]
RC455.4.R4P76   1986   291.1'75   85-28728
ISBN 0-88048-099-8 (soft : alk. paper)

Contents

Contributors

RUTH TIFFANY BARNHOUSE, M.D., TH.M.
Professor of Psychiatry and Pastoral Care, Perkins School of Theology,
Southern Methodist University, Dallas, Texas

DAN G. BLAZER, M.D., PH.D.
Associate Professor of Psychiatry, Director, Division of Social and Community
Psychiatry, Duke University Medical Center, Durham, North Carolina

GALA S. DURRANCE, M.ED.
Executive Director, Be Whole, Orlando, Florida

KLAUS HOPPE, M.D., PH.D.
Associate Professor of Clinical Psychiatry, University of California at Los
Angeles; and Director of Research and Continuing Education,
The Hacker Clinic, Los Angeles, California

BERTON H. KAPLAN, PH.D.
Professor of Epidemiology, The School of Public Health,
University of North Carolina, Chapel Hill, North Carolina

JAMES A. KNIGHT, M.D., B.D., M.P.H.
Professor of Psychiatry and Medical Ethics; and Acting Chairman,
Department of Psychiatry, Louisiana State University School of Medicine,
New Orleans, Louisiana

DAVID B. LARSON, M.D., M.S.P.H.
Research Psychiatrist, Biometric and Clinical Applications Branch, Division of
Biometry and Applied Sciences, National Institute of Mental Health; and
Assistant Professor of Psychiatry, Duke University Medical Center,
Durham, North Carolina

ABDUL R. OMRAN, M.D., D.P.H.
Professor of Epidemiology, The School of Public Health,
University of North Carolina, Chapel Hill, North Carolina

E. MANSELL PATTISON, M.D.
Professor and Chairman, Department of Psychiatry,
Medical College of Georgia, Augusta, Georgia

LILLIAN H. ROBINSON, M.D.

Professor of Psychiatry and Pediatrics; and Training and Supervising Analyst, Analytic Medicine Program, Department of Psychiatry and Neurology, Tulane University School of Medicine, New Orleans, Louisiana

LEON SALZMAN, M.D.

Clinical Professor of Psychiatry, Georgetown University School of Medicine, Washington, DC

SIDNEY WERKMAN, M.D.

Professor of Psychiatry, University of Colorado School of Medicine, Denver, Colorado

Introduction

Healing and religion have been separated only for a few centuries. Consequently it is not surprising that we find parallels in the theoretical systems of dynamic psychiatry and religion, and mutual concerns among their helping professionals. These are explained in this monograph, which grew out of a symposium with the same title presented at the 138th Annual Meeting of the American Psychiatric Association as a joint session of the American Academy of Psychoanalysis and the APA.

Some of the material in Chapters 1 and 2 has been adapted from a previously published paper, "The Illusion of No Future: Psychoanalysis and Religion," which appeared in the *Journal of the American Academy of Psychoanalysis* 13:211–228, 1985. I wish to thank John Wiley and Sons for permission to adapt this material for publication in this monograph. Chapter 1 is a comparison of psychoanalysis and religion, addressing their continuing relevance in our changing world. Chapter 2 is a discussion of advantages gained through collaboration between therapists and clergy.

James Knight, M.D., a psychiatrist and Methodist minister, applies the concept of the *wounded healer* to both disciplines in Chapter 3, and demonstrates the priestly mission of the physician and the healing mission of the minister in Chapter 4.

Leon Salzman, M.D., in Chapter 5, and Ruth Tiffany Barn-house, M.D., in Chapter 6, present their views about the function of religion. Dr. Salzman, in his discussion of the misuse of religion by seriously disturbed patients, states that the function of religion is to provide a feeling of being in control. Dr. Barnhouse agrees that some people use religion in this way but points out that a far more important and appropriate function of religion is to provide cosmic orientation. Dr. Barnhouse, who is both a psychiatrist and an Episcopal priest, provides helpful guidelines for evaluating pa-tients' religious ideation.

The authors of Chapters 7 and 8 were discussants for the sympo-sium papers. Sidney Werkman, M.D., in Chapter 7, notes shared qualities and differences of psychotherapies and religion and dis-cusses religious elements in psychotherapies. In Chapter 8, Klaus Hoppe, M.D., speculates about the future dialogue of psychiatry and religion, as influenced by new discoveries about brain func-tions and neuropsychology. Dr. Hoppe has incorporated in this chapter portions of his paper, "Mind and Spirituality: Symbol-lexia, Empathy, and God-Representation," which was published in Volume 31 of the Bulletin of the National Guild of Catholic Psychiatrists, Inc. Permission from the editor to use the material is gratefully acknowledged.

The two remaining chapters were presented in another sympo-sium at the APA meeting. E. Mansell Pattison, M.D., and Gala S. Durrance, M.Ed., in Chapter 9 report findings of a study of individ-uals who had participated in a religious self-help-group movement in an effort to change from a homosexual to a heterosexual ori-entation. Dr. Pattison is an ordained minister as well as a psychia-trist, and Ms. Durrance is the executive director of Be Whole, an ex-Gay counseling center. David Larson, M.D., and his co-authors, E. Mansell Pattison, M.D., Dan G. Blazer, M.D., Abdul R. Omron, M.D., and Berton H. Kaplan, Ph.D., report in Chapter 10 on their study of the extent to which psychiatric research assesses the role of religion in the lives of psychiatric patients.

I am grateful to Myron Glucksman, M.D., for suggesting that I organize a symposium on this subject; to Ian Alger, M.D., for his advice and participation; and to my husband, Earl W. Robinson, M.D., for his support and forbearance. Finally, I wish to thank the contributors, whose interest in the interfaces of psychiatry and religion made this monograph possible.

Lillian H. Robinson, M.D.

1

Psychoanalysis and Religion: A Comparison

Lillian H. Robinson, M.D.

1

Psychoanalysis and Religion: A Comparison

Medicine and religion have been separated only for a few centuries. It is therefore not surprising that we find many parallels when we compare the theoretical systems of psychoanalysis and religion and the concerns of the helping professionals in each discipline. I will first attempt to explore some of the intriguing similarities and disparities of psychoanalysis and religion, particularly the Judeo-Christian tradition, and then discuss changes each is making in order to remain viable.

COMPARISONS

Psychoanalysis is not yet 100 years old, whereas religion is as old as recorded history, and probably as old as man. Religion seeks an understanding of man's relationship to God and the universe; psychoanalysis is perhaps man's greatest effort to understand man. There are many theologies and metapsychologies which provide useful theoretical frameworks for these inquiries into the nature of God and man. Man's concept of God is constantly changing, despite the efforts of fundamentalist theologians to preserve certain concepts as concrete, absolute truths. Man's understanding of man is also dynamic and evolving, although there are those who adhere rigidly to outmoded concepts. In comparing Christian theology with depth psychology, Ulanov (1) states, "Theology's concern is soteriological; it relates the categories of being to the quest for 'the new being.' Depth psychology is phenomenological; it observes and classifies psychic phenomena in relation to the psychotherapeutic task of healing psychic disturbances" (p. 7). Fromm (2) described a core of ideas and norms common to the teachings of Lao-tse, Buddha, the Prophets, Socrates, Jesus, Spinoza, and the philosophers of the enlightenment: "Man must strive to recognize the truth and can be fully human only to the extent to which he succeeds in this task. He must be independent and free, an end in himself and not the means for any other person's purposes. He must relate himself to his fellow men lovingly. ... Man must know the difference between good and evil, he must learn to listen to the voice of his conscience and to be able to follow it" (p. 76). Fromm added that the aim of psychoanalytic therapy is to help the patient attain this "religious" attitude.

The founder of psychoanalysis did not have a religious upbringing and he professed no religious faith, yet religion fascinated him, and his creation, psychoanalysis, has many aims and values in common with the Jewish and Christian religions. For example, Freud's concept of normality was based on adaptive functioning— the ability to work and to love, which we now extend to include the ability to play. Most religions also place a high value on these activities.

The Bible is a history of people at work (3). Six days of labor are commanded and idleness is disparaged (4–6). In keeping with Hebrew tradition, which required every boy to learn a trade, Jesus learned carpentry from his father. Paul, a hard worker himself, urged his fellow Christians to work and earn their own livings (7, 8). He admonished the church in Thessalonika to ostracize any of its members who refused to work, and reminded them of the rule: "those who don't work, don't eat" (9). It seems that, like today, there were those who just wanted to sit around and wait for the end of the world. Biblical women drudged at grain mills, hearths, with their brooms, at their looms, and with their water jars (10–14). They were shepherdesses, gleaners like Ruth, and businesswomen like Lydia (15–17).

The Bible does not encourage play quite as strongly as work; however, a weekly day of rest is mandated, and Jesus invited discouraged workers to the refreshing rest to be found in spiritual activities: "Come to me, all you who labor and are overburdened and I will give you rest" (18). He also sanctioned wedding feasts and even provided wine for the wedding at Cana (19). Since the Reformation, many Protestant Christian sects have regarded as sinful almost anything that is pleasurable. The Koran is more definite about permission to play. In it we find "man shall be held accountable for all permissible pleasures he fails to enjoy."

Children's play is an important concern of child analysts and child psychiatrists, who regard the ability to enjoy play as an important index of mental health. Erikson (20) referred to play as the work of early childhood. He stated: "[Children's] play . . . is a function of the ego, an attempt to synchronize the bodily and the social processes with the self . . . The child's play . . . [represents] ability to deal with experience by creating model situations and to master reality by experiment and planning" (p. 211). Play can be a means of communicating and an effective medium for therapy of children.

Adults also have a continuing need for play and playfulness. Erikson (20) explained that adult play is different from childhood play. Its function is recreation—"The playing adult steps sideways into another reality; the playing child advances forward to new stages of mastery" (p. 222). Some of our anhedonic patients make no effort to play, whereas others engage in poorly controlled, frantic, pleasure-seeking efforts. Successful analysis frees people to secure pleasure in appropriate ways and modifies the neurotic guilt which is often associated with enjoyment of the "permissible pleasures." Such lifting of the inhibition to play can make life bearable for those who experience their pain and suffering as too great a price to pay for the gratification they can hope to achieve.

The ability to love is considered an ideal quality in the Judeo-Christian tradition. The Ten Commandments provide ground rules for relationships with God and human beings. Unfairness, destructiveness, and lack of respect for others are prohibited. In the religions of primitive people, God is often perceived as harsh and vengeful. Awe and fear are the primary emotional responses to these primitive concepts of God. Doubts about God's goodness are still around, and not just in primitive cultures. In an essay in *The American Scholar*, Furnas (21) cites some of the ironies of life and speculates about the possibility that God may be an unfeeling practical joker who enjoys playing tricks and experimenting with us, much the same way that children enjoy placing twigs in the path of ants, to see whether they will climb over or go around. He quotes Graham Greene, who suggests that "perhaps the dark side of God has a sense of humor." However, in the end, Furnas rejects the notion that "it is irony . . . that makes the world go round" on the grounds that it is too logical to be true. In his words, "nothing that fits the data so well, but is incapable of demonstration, could conceivably be valid" (p. 82).

The Jewish and Christian religions are unique in their emphasis on the reciprocal love between God and humanity. In the Old Testament we find the command to love God with all one's being, and to love our neighbor as we love ourselves (22, 23). Thus, self-esteem is accepted as natural and desirable. In psychoanalysis, the restoration of the analysand's capacity for self-esteem and self-respect is often a therapeutic gain. As overly perfectionistic attitudes and expectations for self and others are relinquished, there is marked improvement in patients' capacities for forming caring relationships. According to Fromm (2), "Analytic therapy is essentially an attempt to help the patient gain or regain his capacity for love" which Fromm defined as "a capacity for the experience of concern, responsibility, respect, and understanding of another person and the intense desire for that other person's growth" (p. 87).

Psychoanalysis and religion have restorative functions and are seen as sources of help in humanity's quest for the good life; both are expected to provide solutions for problems in living and to help people cope with life's vicissitudes. The "examined life" of the religious individual parallels the insight and self-awareness gained through psychoanalysis.

Although spiritual direction and dynamic psychotherapy can be shown to have much in common, psychiatry, including psychoanalysis, is often regarded as an adversary of religion, particularly in cases where religion assumes the role of a harsh superego, opposed to instinctual gratifications. Some religious counselors mistake neurotic guilt for realistic, existential guilt, just as some psychoanalysts with little understanding of religion mistake healthy religious feelings for neurosis. Barnhouse (24) compares the struggle between religion and psychiatry to a custody fight of divorcing parents, and recommends "joint custody" as the best option, pointing out that humankind needs both salvation and healing, and arguing that the two are etymologically as well as fundamentally identical. In her opinion, spiritual directors over-emphasize willpower and have not, until recently, been interested in why and how mistakes and wrong choices are made (25). She quotes the poet, Kahlil Gibran, who said, "The mad man is no less a musician than you or myself; only the instrument on which he plays is a little out of tune" (p. 6), and suggests that, with this metaphor for life, the therapist is the instrument tuner and the spiritual director is the music teacher. We "instrument tuners" don't choose the music or decide how it will be played, but we help get the instrument in shape so the patient can play.

The spiritual director is trained to guide people in their search for values and meaning in life; psychoanalysts are trained to help resolve conflict and achieve a mature adaptation to life. However, when there is conflict about values, the psychoanalyst can help. In his discussion of psychoanalysis and moral values, Hartmann (26) points out that Freud "took pains to keep clinical apart from moral valuation" (p. 17) and stated emphatically that "although . . . psychoanalysis . . . has had great influence on our civilization in . . . moral matters, [Freud's] position as to attempts . . . to deduce a philosophy of life from analysis was unequivocally negative" (p. 20). Jung (27), one of the first to insist that psychoanalysis cannot be value free, stressed the need for analysts to be aware of their own value systems in order to avoid imposing them on their patients. He associated healthy psychological development with religious growth. Acceptance, reconciliation, and strengthening of relationships can result from involvement in psychoanalysis or from religious influences and experiences. Pattison (28) reminds us, on the other hand, that while compliance with religious beliefs, attitudes, and practices can be a powerful force for human good, it can also result in inhuman destructiveness with immature, seriously disturbed individuals. He points out that a religious system assimilated into a primitive superego produces compliance that is not necessarily related to internalized moral values and behavior, whereas a religious system assimilated into mature ego functioning can produce highly ethical behavior.

Barnhouse (25) recalls that many of the discoveries and techniques of psychotherapy have been used by generations of spiritual leaders. For example, St. Ignatius of Loyola, the founder of the Jesuits, understood that in order to be effective, the spiritual director must be able to establish a good rapport with the individual who is seeking help. Another example of similar technique (although for different reasons) is that the priest hearing confessions and the psychoanalyst conducting analysis are traditionally situated outside the visual field of the individuals with whom they are working. The analyst is trying not to be a distraction to the patient, whereas the priest is seeking to preserve the penitent's anonymity.

Both religion and psychoanalysis make use of ritual. Wood (29) has discussed both the constructive and neurotic aspects of ritual. He states that, on the positive side, ritual "provides a constant context within which it becomes safe to explore the inconstant aspects of life, conflict and contradiction" (p. 17). Examples given are the yearly cycle of the reading of the Torah, the Christian liturgical year, and regular analytic sessions within a constant analytic atmosphere and setting. He quotes Vallmerhausen, who warns that although the symbolic system that we use in psychoanalysis helps us organize data, it can also act "like a pair of blinders, obscuring any possibility of seeing the unfamiliar, the unexpected, the peripheral" (p. 17). Wood states that healthy ritual is adaptable and thus enables us to meet the unique needs of our patients: for example, with regard to frequency of sessions, use of the couch, and length of analysis.

Religion and psychoanalysis are both concerned with human anxieties. Anxiety regarding the human condition and the transitory nature of life may be considered primarily a theological concern; neurotic anxiety is the province of psychiatry and psy-choanalysis. There is overlap, however, between neurosis and sin. Horney (30) described the perfectionistic, omnipotent neurotic as the antithesis of the truly religious person, who accepts his or her human limitations. Religion addresses the three existential anxi-eties described by Tillich: anxiety concerning death, the anxiety of meaninglessness, and the anxiety of guilt and condemnation (31). Theologians combat these anxieties, which stem from the nature of man, by assisting with the search for the ultimate courage to be, and to affirm one's self in spite of the threat of nonbeing. Belief in an omnipotent God appears to be a fundamental human need. Voltaire referred to this basic human need of mankind to believe in a power which transcends our personal experience when he stated, "If there were no God, man would have had to invent him." Freud thought man *had* invented God. He regarded faith in God to be an immature clinging to a dependent role and a reluc-tance to relinquish magic. In "The Future of an Illusion," Freud (32) explained his view that religious belief is actually hope, de-rived from man's wish for a solution for helplessness in the face of internal and external dangers, including death. Prentiss Dunn, in an unpublished manuscript, maintains that what Freud attacked as religion is, in reality, "the abuse of religion by individuals who flee to it as a shelter from the realities of a seemingly erratic and impersonal universe that threatens their security and fragile self-esteem."

Some religions promise immortality to the good and the faith-ful. Life on earth is regarded as a temporary state and the eternal afterlife is considered more important. The expectation of immor-tality *should* eliminate some of the death anxiety; however, in view of the fact that death represents an experience of separation as well as a change of status, it is anxiety-provoking even to believers. Also, unfortunately, the human mind tends to have trouble accepting ideas which cannot be proved. Thus the "faith" of many devoutly religious individuals does appear to be predomi-nantly "hope," with only a modicum of conviction. They pray as did the father of the epileptic child, "Lord, I believe; help Thou mine unbelief" (33). Since perfect faith is as impossible for humans as unambivalent love, even the believers among us could be regarded as "a little bit agnostic." Our doubts probably stimulate us to find other avenues to immortality just in case there is no life after death. Pollock (34) states that revolutionaries and believers in artistic, social, political, and scientific causes "feel they can achieve immortality through the permanence of what they value, espouse, and idealize." He suggests further that "one of the motivating stimuli for creativity may be the wish for immortality for the individual and for his product" (p. 348).

Is psychoanalysis different from religion in that it is a science, as Freud, Jung, and many other early analysts regarded it to be? In addressing this question, Salzman (35) stated, "Psychoanalysts are on both sides of the controversy; some emphasize its scientific methodology while others . . . stress . . . the intuitive and artistic elements in psychoanalytic theory and practice." He warned that "by . . . forcing psychoanalysis into the mold of the physical sciences, we may distort and negate its peculiar character as a science which makes subjectivity its main concern" (pp. 5, 6). As analysts we respond defensively to the prevailing view in our culture that only the physical sciences, mathematical in framework and statistically verifiable, merit serious study. We strive to be as objective as possible and tend to be apologetic about the essentially subjective nature of our work, even though we accept the impossibility and undesirability of complete objectivity and neutrality on the part of any therapist. Salzman suggested that in developing "our behavioral science of psychodynamics" we must accept the difficulties in collecting and quantifying data, the impossibility of complete control of variables, and the scarcity of measuring apparatus which could enable us to validate our hypotheses. Rather than attempting to conform to traditional scientific methodology, he recommended that we address ourselves to the development of suitable techniques for handling the data we can obtain, keeping in mind the importance of values as determinants of behavior. On the other hand, Earl Witenberg (36) maintained that psychoanalysis is not a science, inasmuch as its theories, which "attempt to give meaning to . . . behavior, thinking, affects, imagery, development and . . . the unconscious" (p. 433), are essentially belief systems, originated by one individual on the basis of observations of patients. He ascribed efforts to make a science out of psychoanalysis, by scientifically proving its theories, to our need to believe in a higher authority. Barnhouse (24) has also argued that psychoanalysis is not a science but a metaphysical system, like religion. She attributes psychiatry's "superiority complex vis-a-vis religion" (p. 12) to the assumption that it is scientific and she warns that "remedicalization of psychiatry may cause unique psychological events to be overlooked . . . [since] that which cannot be measured gets ignored when people are too firmly wedded to the scientific mind-set" (p. 14).

There seems to be general agreement as to the impossibility of proving the validity of psychoanalytic theory by experimental means. There is also agreement on the improbability of making accurate predictions about multidetermined human behavior, and there is consensus that it is futile to try to prove the efficacy of psychoanalysis by research methods which take it out of its natural context, and perhaps distort it. In the final analysis, we can think of psychoanalysis as a science with challenging research difficulties or take the position that, although it is not science in the strict sense, it utilizes another approach to valid knowledge.

The sticking point appears to be the definition of science. In Webster's Collegiate Dictionary, fourth edition, we find, "science is systematized knowledge considered in reference to the discovery of understanding of truth; art is knowledge as applied and made efficient by skill. If, then, a body of laws and principles . . . is exhibited in an ordered and interrelated system, they appear in the character of a science. If they are applied in actual use, they become, or furnish the working rules of, an art." According to these definitions, it would appear that psychoanalysis is an art and can also be a science, as long as we retain a scientific, questioning, searching attitude which avoids our becoming so enamored of a theory that we cannot accept evidence that refutes it. We must constantly modify theory in accord with new data. Many psychoanalytic concepts, including ego, id, superego, defense mechanisms, and the unconscious, are neither provable nor refutable. Their scientific merit depends not on provable validity, but on their organizing qualities and heuristic value. They are not observable facts, but provide a conceptual framework useful for the study and understanding of human behavior.

The ideological systems of psychoanalysis and religion, though different, are not necessarily incompatible. Religion is based on faith in God and concerns itself with values; psychoanalysis is based on faith in people's ability to change. Arieti (37) said it eloquently: "Neither despair nor pessimism will prevail if [we] feel that it is never too late in life to correct past mistakes. Until his last breath, the human being can grow, can innovate, and to some extent, with the help of others he can create his life" (p. 184). Theologians share this belief. They regard the creative potential for change to be a God-given quality which makes repentance and amendment of life a possibility. Knight (38) has suggested that "cooperative efforts of psychiatry and religion may well result in helping modern man find answers to some of his crucial questions on his predicament" (p. 30). These cooperative efforts have increased in recent years. Knowledge of psychodynamics has enabled the clergy to understand neurotic guilt and has contributed to their counseling skills; many clergy make appropriate referrals to psychiatrists and psychoanalysts. Unfortunately, few psychiatrists or analysts recognize those cases who could benefit from consultation with a spiritual advisor.

Another feature common to psychoanalysis and religion is that both are in crisis, struggling to remain relevant and meaningful in our changing world. Two decades ago the value of both religion and psychoanalysis was beginning to be questioned by many. A *Time Magazine* cover story addressed the "rumor" that God is dead, and advances in psychopharmacology led some psychiatrists to conclude that psychoanalysis had outlined its usefulness.

Cox (39) has traced the evolution of present trends in religion. He states that modern theology emerged "out of a cultural milieu in which religion was in retreat and skepticism seemed to be gaining on every hand. The 'project' of modern theology was to make faith credible once again to the intellectual pace setters who were leaving it behind. ... As what has been called the 'post modern' era begins, it is not religion but the modern world itself

which is threatened with oblivion" (p. 3). In Cox's opinion modern theology addresses itself to the group designated by Schleier-
macher as the *cultured despisers* of religion; post-modern religion
is action oriented and addresses the condition and needs of the
despised. Cox suggests that "we need a post-modern theology in
order to cope not with the decline of religion but with its resur-
gence; not with the death of God but with the rebirth of Gods . . ."
(p. 3). The trend in religion now is to concentrate more on the
social significance of theological ideas rather than on theology
itself. Post-modern religion pursues social and political activism in
order to counteract oppression and discrimination. Cox cautions
that, in order to succeed, the new theology must not discard the
brilliant insights of modern theology but must incorporate them.

Franzblau's (40) description of *mature religion* seems relevant to
a post-modern theology. He defines mature religions as those
which "do not foster neurotic mechanisms in the worshipper but
make for soundness and health in mind, spirit and values . . . they
are man-fostering rather than man-flagellating; their concern is
man's ultimate worth, not his original sin; they advocate a robust
morality in the sexual realm rather than an ascetic code; . . . their
ethics are deed-centered rather than creed-centered; they foster
aggressiveness in the face of evil, rather than a supine passivity;
their guilt concept is not ecclesiogenic, but is related to reality;
they eschew fear of punishment in this world or the next, or the
promise of reward as motivations for good behavior; their major
emphasis is this-worldly, rather than other-worldly, progressivis-
tic, rather than perfectionistic . . ." (p. 124).

I agree with those who propose that psychiatry today is faced
with a similar need to retain the old while embracing the new.
Dynamic psychiatry, like modern theology, is much too valuable
to be discarded as anachronistic and useless. Regarding the value of
psychoanalysis, Wood (29) suggests that the Biblical test of grace/
health 'By their fruits you shall know them' can be applied and if
psychoanalysis leads to deeper and more compassionate connections with self and others, in the past, present, and future, it is a
constructive process. Pollock has speculated that "the survival and
flowering of our science of man may, in the long run, be our most

significant contribution and the application of this science to the therapeutic situation may be of lesser importance" (41, p. 29). Psychoanalytic theory has contributed significantly to all fields involving human psychological functioning, including social and biological sciences, the humanities, theology, law, and medicine. It is so much a part of psychiatry that many psychiatrists are not aware of the psychoanalytic origin of certain concepts they use every day. In one survey of psychiatrists, the majority stated that psychoanalytic concepts were not useful in psychiatric practice. When asked what they did regard as useful, many of these same psychiatrists said they found the concept of defense mechanisms to be quite valuable! I agree with Hawkins that "the dynamic viewpoint is well established in American academic psychiatry and is generally well integrated with the biological viewpoint, particularly in research centers" (42, p. 715).

Psychoanalytic influence has also greatly benefitted other medical specialties, by promoting a more holistic and humanistic approach to patients. The findings of analysts who have directly observed the effects on infants of illness and hospitalization have led to changes in the primary-care physician's understanding of the needs of sick children. These analysts, often working in medical school departments of psychiatry, have made valuable contributions to the care of sick children through applications of their research.

Spitz (43), for example, began systematic observations of infants in 1935, which led to his discovery that severe depression and "arrest in the development of all sectors of the personality" can result from early loss and inadequate replacement of the mothering person (p. 285). He demonstrated that physical care, without a relationship with the caregiver, cannot compensate for this loss because of the infant's need for a steady, reciprocating, caring person whose style becomes consistently manifest in the life of the infant.

Anna Freud and Burlingham (44), in discussing work with war orphans and infants temporarily separated from their parents because of the bombings in London, provided additional evidence that disruption of early relationships is a developmental interference that can lead to severe regressions and problems in forming relationships. Bowlby (45), Robertson (46), Prugh et al. (47), and Solnit (48) have observed the effects of short separations from parents incidental to a young child's hospitalization. Their work added to our understanding of the nature and intensity of the stress of illness, hospitalization, and surgery; the immature ego's attempts at coping; and the role of parents in lending ego support to children in these situations.

These and other careful observational studies have gradually led to changes in hospital policies regarding parental visiting. It was often assumed formerly that, since children were less trouble and could be managed more easily alone, it was preferable to exclude parents, especially when frightening or painful procedures needed to be carried out. Parents are now encouraged to spend as much time as possible with their hospitalized infants and young children, to help in their care, and especially to be present to support and reassure their children during frightening procedures.

Analytic studies have contributed much understanding about the importance to a child's mental health of good child–parent relationships. Fernholt and Provence (49) demonstrated that infants who develop "in the climate of a profound disturbance in the mother–child relationship . . . suffer from deficits and distortions of the protective, the stimulating, and the organizing aspects of parental care" (p. 455). This failure of the auxiliary ego can manifest itself as a psychophysiological disturbance, such as colic or vomiting, or in the failure-to-thrive syndrome.

Fraiberg and associates (50) developed innovative programs, going to the homes to help young parents who had been abused or deprived in early life and who were therefore at risk for abusing and depriving their own babies. The parents learned to enjoy caring for their infants and to be responsive to their signals and needs. The helping teams enabled the parents to get in touch with feelings about childhood difficulties with their own parents and to resolve some of the old conflicts which were interfering with their parenting. Often they learned to treat their children the way they would have wished their parents to treat them, instead of duplicating their own parents' negligent or abusive behavior.

These are but a few of the many examples of beneficial effects of psychoanalytic input to the care of children. Many other aspects of patient care, including the management of the dying patient and preventive interventions for individuals in crisis situations, have also been greatly influenced by analytic thought. Much of the psychiatric input to other medical specialties in consultation/liaison services is based on psychodynamic understanding of patients' feelings about their illnesses—feelings which are sometimes expressed through disruptive or uncooperative behavior, which can be managed better when it is understood.

During the last two decades, however, many psychiatrists, who were becoming disenchanted with psychoanalysis because they had expected too much from it, turned to the emerging field of biological psychiatry, and expected too much from psychopharmacology. Psychiatry can usefully retain dynamic understanding as it seeks more effective drugs and more knowledge about the neurochemical correlates of behavior. Biological psychiatrists and psychoanalysts can each avail themselves of the contributions of the other for the benefit of their patients. Several analysts, including Anna Freud (51), have reported favorable results with the combination of psychoanalysis and drug therapy for depressed patients. Spiegel (52) advocates more use of a variety of therapies (including drugs, group, family or conjoint marital therapy, biofeedback, meditation, behavior therapy, and so forth) in conjunction with psychoanalysis, particularly when little progress is being made with psychoanalysis alone. The following vignette is illustrative:

A 41-year-old woman college professor began analysis because of recurrent episodes of depression, problems with important relationships, severe recurrent headaches, and functional gastrointestinal disturbances. As a child she had worried a great deal about her mother, who had a chronic physical illness and was often depressed. She had idealized her father but also had resented him when her mother grieved about his many affairs. The patient gained a great deal of self understanding, and became able to relate in a warmer, more-accepting way to others, as she freed herself from maladaptive reaction patterns belonging to the past, but

somatic symptoms continued to be troublesome. After biofeedback was added, her physical symptoms gradually subsided. An
earlier course of biofeedback training, prior to her beginning analysis, had not been effective.

Of course it is impossible to know whether the same good result
could have been achieved by persevering with psychoanalysis
alone; however, the two approaches seemed to be complementary
and the combination was probably speedier and more cost effective in reaching a resolution of her problem than if either had
been used singly. It is important to design treatment plans that
meet the individual needs of the particular patient rather than to
expect the patient to fit our preferred therapeutic modality.

In recent decades, analysts have become increasingly concerned
about the confusion and conflict in their field, which could
threaten the survival and continuing usefulness of psychoanalysis.
Many have advocated closer cooperation between analytic groups
of Freudians, Jungians, neo-Freudians, and others, to work toward
resolution of conflicting views about theory, training, and practice, and to join in research efforts to study the results of psychoanalytic treatment.

Despite the fact that conducting a psychoanalysis is essentially a
joint research project, in which the patient supplies the data and
the analyst provides the expertise for understanding the data,
psychoanalysts are not necessarily effective researchers in the classical sense. Shakow (53) observed that many of the physicians who
are attracted to psychoanalysis are primarily interested in clinical
work and lack a research outlook and motivation. Pollock (41)
decried the isolation of psychoanalysis from the rest of medicine,
the arts, the humanities, and the biological and social sciences and
stated that "psychoanalytic clinicians alone may not be the researchers we need to further our science" (p. 25). Continuing
development of psychoanalytic theory is dependent upon continuing research and scholarship. If we become completely absorbed in
its clinical application, there is danger that its development as a
basic science will be neglected. A safeguard which should insure
against such an eventuality would be to base psychoanalytic training increasingly in universities, the institutions in our society

whose function is to encourage scholarship and research.

In order to ensure the ongoing usefulness of psychiatry and psychoanalysis, we must learn to synthesize old knowledge with new, and utilize opportunities to choose new directions. The goal of continuity is best achieved through an ongoing process, open to change. This is the challenge we are facing and it is up to us, individually and collectively, to respond.

References

1. Ulanov AB: The Feminine in Jungian Psychology and in Christian Theology. Evanston, IL, Northwestern University Press, 1971

2. Fromm E: Psychoanalysis and Religion. New Haven, Yale University Press, 1950

3. Miller MS, Miller JL: The New Harper's Bible Dictionary. New York, Harper and Row, 1973

4. Exodus 34:21

5. Proverbs 6:6–11

6. Proverbs 24:30–34

7. Acts 18:3

8. I Thessalonians 4:11

9. II Thessalonians 3:6–11

10. Matthew 24:41

11. Genesis 18:6

12. Luke 15:8

13. I Samuel 2:19

14. Genesis 24:15

15. Genesis 29:6

16. Ruth 2:13

17. Acts 16:14

18. Matthew 11:28-30

19. John 2:1-11

20. Erikson EH: Childhood and Society. New York, WW Norton, 1950

21. Furnas JE: The ant and the twig; or, the dark side of God. The American Scholar 53:63-82, 1983

22. Deuteronomy 6:4

23. Leviticus 19:18

24. Barnhouse RT: Psychiatry and religion: partners or strangers? Paper presented at the Annual Meeting of the American Academy of Psychoanalysis, New York, December, 1981

25. Barnhouse RT: Spiritual direction and psychotherapy. Trinity News 30:6-7, 15, 1983

26. Hartmann H: Psychoanalysis and Moral Values. New York, International Universities Press, 1960

27. Jung C: Psychology and Religion. New Haven, Yale University Press, 1938

28. Pattison EM: Religion and compliance, in Compliant Behavior: Beyond Obedience to Authority. Edited by Rosenbaum M. New York, Human Sciences Press, 1983

29. Wood BG: The religion of psychoanalysis. Am J Psychoanal 40:13-22, 1981

30. Horney K: Neurosis and Human Growth. New York, WW Norton, 1950

31. Tillich P: The Courage to Be. New Haven, Yale University Press, 1952

32. Freud S: The Future of an Illusion (1927), in Complete Psychological Works, Standard Edition, vol. 21. Translated and edited by Strachey J. London, Hogarth Press, 1961

33. Mark 9:24

34. Pollock GH: On mourning, immortality, and utopia. J Am Psychoanal Assoc 23:334-362, 1975

35. Salzman L: Presidential address: psychoanalysis and science, in Science and Psychoanalysis, vol. 9. Edited by Masserman J. New York, Grune & Stratton, 1966

36. Witenberg EG: Presidential address: to believe or not to believe. J Am Acad Psychoanal 4:433-445, 1976

37. Arieti S: Presidential address: psychoanalytic therapy in a cultural climate of pessimism. J Am Acad Psychoanal 9:171-184, 1981

38. Knight JA: A Psychiatrist Looks at Religion and Health. New York, Abingdon Press, 1964

39. Cox H: Religion in the secular city. Ministry Development Journal 4:3-8, 1984

40. Franzblau AN: Discussion of Apolito's "Psychoanalysis and religion." Am J Psychoanal 30:123-126, 1970

41. Pollock G: The mourning process and creative organizational change. J Am Psychoanal Assoc 25:3-34, 1977

42. Hawkins DR: Impressions of psychiatric education in Western European specialty training. Arch Gen Psychiatry 36:713-717, 1979

43. Spitz R: The First Year of Life. New York, International Universities Press, 1965

44. Freud A, Burlingham D: War and Children. New York, International Universities Press, 1943

45. Bowlby J: Childhood mourning and its implications for psychiatry. Am J Psychiatry 117:481–498, 1961

46. Robertson J: Hospitals and Children: A Parent's Eye View. New York, International Universities Press, 1962

47. Prugh DG, Staub EM, Sands HH, et al: A study of the emotional reactions of children and families to hospitalization and illness. Am J Orthopsychiatry 23:70–106, 1953

48. Solnit AJ: A study of object loss in infancy. Psychoanal Study Child 25:257–272, 1970

49. Fernholt J, Provence S: Diagnosis and treatment of an infant with psychophysiological vomiting. Psychoanal Study Child 31:439–459, 1976

50. Fraiberg S, Adelson E, Shapiro V: Ghosts in the nursery: a psychoanalytic approach to the problems of impaired infant–mother relationships. J Am Acad Child Psychiatry 14:387–421, 1975

51. Freud A: A letter from Anna Freud. Am J Psychiatry 140:1583, 1983

52. Spiegel JP: Presidential address: the future of psychoanalysis. Presented at the Annual Meeting of the American Academy of Psychoanalysis, New York, May 1983

53. Shakow D: Psychoanalytic education of behavioral and social scientists for research, in Science and Psychoanalysis, vol. 5. Edited by Masserman J. New York, Grune & Stratton, 1962

2

Therapist–Clergy Collaboration

Lillian H. Robinson, M.D.

2

Therapist–Clergy Collaboration

Many psychiatrists neglect to deal with religious themes raised by their patients. This is unfortunate in view of the fact that some patients have troublesome conflicts about religion that could probably be resolved through the process of therapy. Apolito (1) has suggested that analysts often have difficulty in dealing with patients' religious conflicts because their own religious conflicts are unresolved. It becomes essential however, for therapists to address religious issues when they are used by the patient as resistance. Collaborating with the patient's spiritual director can be helpful in overcoming this form of resistance. Unfortunately, psychiatrists rarely consider this option. Physicians in other medical specialties seem more aware than psychiatrists of the advantages to be gained from working together with clergy. Advances in medical knowledge have created frightening ethical problems, including those regarding prolongation of life and organ transplantation. Clergy can provide meaningful assistance to those physicians and patients who struggle with these problems. Physicians and the clergy have many mutual concerns, including the concern for wholeness and the alleviation of suffering.

There are probably many reasons why psychiatrists and other mental health professionals have been slow to recognize that they and the clergy often need each other. Barnhouse (2) attributes the condescending attitude of many psychiatrists toward religion partly to the assumption that psychotherapy is a science. She adds, "Furthermore, psychiatry has been extremely critical of the crippling effects which certain kinds of religious belief have had on psychological development, since such effects had often been demonstrated to be a significant etiological factor in psychopathology. Of course, to maintain this critical attitude psychiatric professionals must conveniently ignore the numerous cases in which ill-advised psychiatric techniques have been equally harmful. Religious professionals, on the other hand, have generally felt themselves to be either above or beneath science. Those who feel above it believe that scripture . . . has a higher claim to truth . . . and . . . feel free to discard conclusions of science if these do not . . . cohere with their views. Other religious professionals . . . accept the priority of science, and are willing . . . to discard such portions of their . . . belief as may be demonstrated to conflict with it. Neither attitude—either that of superiority or inferiority—is conducive to any real cooperation between the two disciplines" (pp. 131, 132). Pattison (3) also blames mental health professionals for the lack of "reciprocity of referral back and forth. . . ." He points out that "clergy often are not encouraged by mental health professionals, are treated rudely or with disdain, or ignored . . ." (p. 126).

The literature on the subject includes speculation that psychoanalysts' lack of interest in religion, and reluctance to deal with religious issues in their clinical work, might be due in part to Freud's negative assessment of it. In "Obsessive Actions and Religious Practices," Freud suggested that obsessional neurosis could be regarded as individual religiosity and religion as a universal obsessional neurosis (4). On the other hand, he valued the ethical teachings of the Jewish religion, and although he regarded Christianity to be a regression rather than a progression, he was, at times, respectful and tolerant of it. In one of his letters to Pfeister, the Swiss cleric, he spoke enthusiastically about the complementary relationship psychoanalysis and religion could have: "people do not come to a physician expecting moral elevation . . . but you are in the fortunate position of leading them on to God. . . . In itself, psychoanalysis is neither religious nor the opposite but an impersonal instrument which can serve the clergy as well as the laity when it is used only to free suffering people. I have been very struck at realizing how I'd never thought of the extraordinary help the psychoanalytic method can be in pastoral work, probably because wicked heretics like us are so far away from that circle" (5, pp. 16, 17). In "The Future of an Illusion" (6), he expressed the opinion that religion "arose out of the Oedipus complex, out of the relation to the father" and stated "if this view is right it is to be supposed that a turning away from religion is bound to occur with . . . the process of growth . . . but I will moderate my zeal and admit the possibility that I too am chasing an illusion" (pp. 43, 48). Using the device of a debate with an imaginary adversary, he then advanced some powerful arguments that religion is useful, practical, and needed as a "basis of education and of man's communal life" (p. 52). In "Civilization and its Discontents" (7), he referred to religion as mental infantilism which induces mass delusion but added that it "spares many people an individual neurosis" (p. 85).

It seems clear that Freud was intrigued with religion and that he recognized its value, even though he disparaged the need for it as "immature." Zilboorg (8) concluded that Freud struggled with unresolved religious conflict and that his vehement denouncements revealed repressed, deeply religious convictions. Apolito (1) suggests that this is also true of many analysts today. Franzblau (9) agreed with this position and quoted a Jewish wit, "nobody ever leaves the synagogue—he only modifies the ritual a bit to suit his individual form of dissent" (p. 125). In discussing *return phenomena*, he cites the example of a psychoanalyst who enrolled his children in a religious school, insisting that he was an atheist, despite this action to the contrary. Two years later the "atheist" had become a member of the board of the synagogue. A survey by the American Psychiatric Association (APA) Committee on Psychiatry and Religion has shown, as one would expect, that most of the psychiatrists who serve religious institutions as consultants, advisors, teachers, or therapists profess to be religious (10). It is Apolito's view that many individuals who proudly flaunt their agnosticism have not really given up belief but have repressed it

(1). He quoted Pruyser, who believes that most people who profess no religion are in reality rebelling against religion. Apolito concludes that "repudiation of the parents' religious and moral values may be the expression of rebellion against the parents rather than a genuine change in beliefs" (pp. 119, 120). This is compatible with the findings of Henry et al. (12) that, although most psychotherapists, from various disciplines, deny having a religious commitment, they usually do come from religious backgrounds.

If it is true that many therapists have unresolved religious conflicts, it seems safe to say that this could render them ineffective in dealing with patients who use religion as a defense and with patients who struggle with religious conflict. It does not seem surprising, therefore, that many therapists either avoid this material or deal with their patients' religious beliefs as though they were pathological. The agnostic therapist might find it difficult to distinguish between healthy, adaptive religious practices and beliefs, and those which are pathological, because of the discrepancy between the orientations of therapist and patient. On the other hand, a shared belief system between patient and therapist can be used by the patient as a means to avoid certain topics and feelings (13). The therapist who shares, or at least respects, patients' beliefs and has no personal conflict about religion may still have difficulty helping patients who confuse existential and neurotic guilt. Collaboration with the patient's spiritual director can be exceedingly helpful in these cases. Although some religious sects foster neurotic guilt in their followers, spiritual directors with whom I have collaborated are sympathetic to my efforts to modify the punitive superegos of individuals for whom religion has assumed this role. On the other hand, some therapists with little understanding of religion are prone to mistake healthy religious feelings for pathological narcissism. Hoppe (14), in distinguishing between them, states, "If a person is capable of cosmic experiences, so quintessentially expressed in Schiller's 'Lied an die Freude' . . . in Beethoven's Ninth Symphony; if emphatically he can sing, 'Brothers, over the tent of stars, a good father must live,' then he cannot be narcissistic. If he is narcissistic, i.e., only idealizing himself, he cannot experience the cosmos" (p. 39). Hoppe proposes that with mature development, including the acquisition of *cosmic empathy*, it becomes possible to achieve the highest level of religious experience, which the Jesuit psychoanalyst, Meissner (15), described as one which integrates empathy, creativity, knowing through faith, selfless love, and acceptance of others. Spiritual directors guide people in their search for values, whereas psychoanalysts and other psychoanalytically oriented therapists try to help them resolve conflict and find their own solutions. When there is conflict about values, the therapist should not hesitate to intercede. Franzblau (9) put it well: "We . . . should accept all manifestations of religion in our patients with respect and objectivity, working not to disillusion . . . but . . . to discover whether they cross the borderline to pathology and interfere with the capacity to function effectively in life. If we . . . discover pathology, our job is to try to cure it. The Church [also] frowns on scrupulosity" (p. 125).

Sevensky (16) describes psychopathological distortions of religion including the inability to feel forgiven, "a syndrome appearing especially among devout, active, and conscientious Christians and taking the form of scrupulosity, . . . intense feelings of unworthiness, the belief that one has committed the unpardonable sin or . . . that one is beyond the love and mercy of God" (p. 81). These patients suffer from obsessional neurosis and are vulnerable to depression. Frequently they are much more impressed by a spiritual director's pronouncement that their "moral issue" is actually a neurotic problem than they are by similar statements made by the therapist. An obsessional man (whose sleeping during sessions was described in an earlier paper) illustrates this quite well (17).

Case Example

J., a 28-year-old accountant, entered analysis because of doubts and fears about his approaching marriage. He had an overly close relationship with his mother, who had never been comfortable away from her own mother. He had always yearned to be able to confide in his father, a devout Roman Catholic who devoted himself to his business and paid little attention to J. except for enforcing discipline. When J.

was five years of age, his father told him that masturbation was sinful and would "ruin" him if he indulged in it. Later on, this was reinforced by the nuns at his Roman Catholic school. When he was 17, he became quite aroused while engaged in heavy petting with a girl and masturbated after taking her home. He felt very guilty, and repeatedly struck his testicles as punishment. He now feared that this may have rendered him sterile or impotent.

J. had attended college for four years but had difficulty making himself study. As soon as he began to be successful he would neglect his assignments until he fell hopelessly behind. He felt embarrassed and self-conscious about not yet having his degree. After a tour of active military service he made several attempts to find a job. Failing in this, he entered seminary, where he remained for four miserable months; then withdrew and joined his father's firm, continuing half-heartedly to pursue his college degree by enrolling in night classes. He began dating a college student, and they became engaged after an 18-month courtship. He attended mass frequently and spent a great deal of time discussing theology and philosophy with Jesuit priests.

On several occasions, with J.'s permission, I conferred with his parish priest, who was also his spiritual director. The priest and I agreed that J.'s religious commitment was sincere and deep, despite his immature and frequently neurotic way of expressing it.

In every session J. reported obsessional thoughts about breaking his engagement, insulting his future in-laws, disrupting the ceremony, or being impotent on his wedding night. He had a fantasy that the wedding had to be postponed because he had forgotten to have the marriage banns published. When he and his fiancée went to the priest to arrange for this to be done, he became quite upset by the question, "Have you ever taken any vows against marriage?" He told the priest that when he entered seminary he had secretly vowed never to marry. The priest explained that this was not a formal vow and therefore was not binding. J. reported this, in his session the following day, and added that he didn't feel reassured and thought it might be a sin to marry because of the secret vow. He said he planned to discuss the matter with another priest, whom he regarded to be stricter. I said I thought, if he shopped around, he probably could find a priest who would say it would be sinful for him to marry. He was somewhat shaken by this, and said he found it hard to believe that he wanted someone to forbid his marriage, as I was implying. It seemed to him that he only wanted to be reassured that it was permissible for him to marry.

A few days later he reported strong urges to return to seminary. He consulted a priest he scarcely knew about his misgivings and was furious because he thought the priest took his feeling that he was being called to the priesthood rather lightly, and also questioned whether he was stable or mature enough for marriage.

As the wedding approached, he reported dreams of having sexual activity with girls other than Linda, his fiancée. He agonized over feeling unfaithful to her because of these dreams. It surprised him to discover that the wishes for other girls occurred when he was attempting to deny that he felt justifiably angry with Linda for some inconsiderate action. He spent many hours trying to decide whether he truly loved her.

The last session before the wedding was painful for J. He cried repeatedly and implored me to tell him what to do. He believed he loved and wanted Linda, but he had strong urges to run away or take to his bed and refuse to go through with the ceremony. After I made an effort to help him understand his opposite wishes, he reported feeling panic-stricken by the thought that he would lose control over his life if he married. I assured him that he would indeed give up a certain amount of control over his future if he married Linda, closing the door forever to the priesthood and to "carefree" bachelorhood. After a thoughtful silence, he stated that this was what he wanted with all his heart, despite his reluctance "to give up any control."

When he returned from his honeymoon, J. reported that his misgivings about getting married had vanished the moment the service began. When he saw Linda coming down the aisle on her father's arm, he experienced only joy and pleasurable anticipation. He regarded the honeymoon to be a real triumph, because he and Linda both enjoyed their first sexual intercourse. His peace of mind was short-lived, however, and he began to talk of his fears that Linda had been or would be unfaithful, eventually coming to understand this as projected self-doubts. He then became preoccupied with the thought that he might be unfaithful to Linda. He felt angry and disappointed because marriage had not solved all his problems. Once when he passed a pretty girl on the street he felt sexually aroused and had a fleeting thought that he would like to make love to her. He then hurried to his priest to confess that he had committed adultery in his heart. The priest said his fantasy was not a sin and suggested that he needed to discuss the guilt with his analyst. His confessor's response made him angry. He went to confession in a different parish and was told that he should consult a psychiatrist.

A few days later, J. reported that he had found a "more respectful" priest, who heard his confession and pronounced absolution without making derogatory remarks about his mental stability. He added that, in spite of this, he still felt very guilty. He had assigned himself extra

prayers in an effort to atone for his sins but when he said the rosary
the idea occurred to him that he had skipped a decade and he felt he
should start over again. This exchange followed:

Patient: I think I lack confidence in myself and feel I can't do anything right. I realize it's extremely unlikely that I would skip a
whole decade in saying the rosary but the thought keeps running
through my mind that I have to get these prayers right in order to
be forgiven, even though the priest pronounced absolution.
Analyst: Why would different rules apply to you than those which
other people live by?
Patient: I have wondered about that . . . I know that if you do something you shouldn't and feel regret and ask forgiveness, that is all
that is supposed to be necessary. I guess it's my wish to be special.
When I was a little boy, my brother was special because of his
handicap and I craved all the extra love and attention which he got.
I kept thinking of how I wanted to be really special and I think I
convinced myself that I am, and that ordinary rules don't apply to
me—that I deserve special dispensations, and that my little sins are
serious crimes, and it seems like I shouldn't get my degree unless I
can graduate summa cum laude. It's pretty grandiose, isn't it? I've
got to convince myself that I can be happy without pretending that
I'm the center of the universe.

Although the nuns in his Catholic school had contributed to
his feeling that sex was dirty and sinful, J.'s spiritual director and
most of the other priests whom he consulted during his analysis
were forthright and confronting in their efforts to help him realize
that his overly scrupulous, perfectionistic expectations for himself
were expressions of an emotional problem rather than legitimate
religious attitudes. Although J. was always very angry when the
priests insisted that he was neurotically scrupulous, he respected
their views, and was sufficiently open-minded to benefit from a
look at his problems from their point of view.

Greenberg (18) has reported receiving similar cooperation from
rabbis who collaborated with him in efforts to help patients with
severe religious compulsions. Pre-prayer ablutions were forbidden
by the rabbis for patients whose handwashing rituals prior to
prayers were extremely lengthy, and repetition of prayers was
banned for those who spent a great deal of time repeating certain

parts over and over, in case mistakes or omissions had occurred.

Although spiritual advisors and psychoanalysts work in different ways, with different goals, both try to bring about change for the better. Barnhouse (1) views both disciplines as *metasystems of reform* and states that "each side has important pieces of the puzzle which could be extremely helpful to the other" (p. 133). A holistic, integrated view of man demands consideration of the physical, the psychological, and the spiritual being. Just as clergy cannot afford to ignore the physical and psychological aspects of man, therapists should not ignore their patients' religious selves. To do so is to overlook a potential source of growth and strength as well as possible repositories of resistance.

REFERENCES

1. Apolito A: Psychoanalysis and religion. Am J Psychoanal 30:115–123, 1970

2. Barnhouse RT: The vicissitudes of reform. Union Seminary Quarterly Review 36:131–140, 1981

3. Pattison EM: Psychiatry and religion circa 1978: analysis of a decade, part II. Pastoral Psychology 27:119–141

4. Freud S: Obsessive Actions and Religious Practices (1907), in Complete Psychological Works, Standard Edition, vol. 9. Translated and edited by Strachey J. London, Hogarth Press, 1959

5. Meng H, Freud E: Psychoanalysis and Faith—The Letters of Sigmund Freud and Oscar Pfister. New York, Basic Books, 1963

6. Freud S: The Future of an Illusion (1927), in Complete Psychological Works, Standard Edition, vol. 21. Translated and edited by Strachey J. London, Hogarth Press, 1961

7. Freud S: Civilization and Its Discontents (1930), in Complete Psychological Works, Standard Edition, vol. 21. Translated and edited by Strachey J. London, Hogarth Press, 1961

8. Zilboorg G: Freud and Religion: A Restatement. London, Geoffrey Chapman, 1958

9. Franzblau AN: Discussion of Apolito's "Psychoanalysis and religion." Am J Psychoanal 30:123–126, 1970

10. Franzblau AN: Psychiatrists' Viewpoints of Religion and Their Services to Religious Institutions and the Ministry. Task Force Report 10. Washington DC, American Psychiatric Association, 1975

11. Pattison EM: Psychiatry and religion circa 1978: analysis of a decade, part I. Pastoral Psychology 27:8–25, 1978

12. Henry WE, Sims JH, Spray SL: The Fifth Profession. San Francisco, Jossey-Bass, 1971

13. Kehoe N, Gutheil TG: Shared religious belief as resistance in psychotherapy. Am J Psychother 38:579–585, 1984

14. Hoppe KD: Psychoanalysis and Christian religion: past views and new findings. Bulletin of the National Guild of Catholic Psychiatrists 30:32–42, 1984

15. Meissner W: Psychoanalytic aspects of religious experience, in The Annual of Psychoanalysis. New York, International Universities Press, 1978

16. Sevensky RL: Religion, psychology, and mental health. Am J Psychother 38:73–86, 1984

17. Robinson LH: Sleep and dreams in the analytic hour: the analysis of an obsessional patient. Psychoanal Rev 61:115–131; 1974

18. Greenberg D: Are religious compulsions religious or compulsive? a phenomenological study. Am J Psychother 38:524–532, 1984

3

The Religio-Psychological Dimension of Wounded Healers

James A. Knight, M.D., B.D., M.P.H.

3

The Religio-Psychological Dimension of Wounded Healers

The physician or priest as healer can be more fully understood when considered in the light of the archetype of the wounded healer. The mythological image of the wounded healer, the myth of Asklepios, proclaims that the patient has a healer within, and the healer a patient within (1). Those in the healing professions (especially physicians and clergy) often give the impression that they are immune to weakness, illness, and wounds, and that patients live in a completely different world. The healers then develop into therapists-without-wounds and can no longer constellate or release the inner healing factor in their patients or themselves.

Carl Jung, in interpreting the Greek myth of the wounded healer, emphasized that "only the wounded doctor can heal, whether that doctor be physician or priest" (p. 116). That is, only the one who is open, sensitive, and *personally* knowledgeable about pain and suffering can participate in healing. One's own hurt, one's sensitive openness to the patient, gives the measure of one's power to heal. Jung's interpretation of the myth of Asklepios, the paradigm of the wounded healer, is generally the way it is seen today (2).

Asklepios, the son of the god Apollo and the mortal woman Koronis, was wounded before birth. Koronis had been unfaithful to Apollo and was shot during her pregnancy by Apollo's sister Artemis, at the instigation of Apollo. While Koronis was on the funeral pyre, Apollo snatched his son Asklepios from her womb, saved him from the flames, and gave him to the healer Chiron to raise and instruct in the art of healing. The myth describes Asklepios's entry into the world as a miraculous birth in death. Chiron, to whom Asklepios was entrusted, was half human and half divine, and afflicted with an incurable wound by the poisoned arrows of Hercules. Thus, Chiron, a healer who needed healing himself, passed on to Asklepios the art of healing, the capacity to be at home in the darkness of suffering and there to find seeds of light and recovery (3, 4).

Another dimension of the wounded healer is that of the suffering servant described in the Book of Isaiah, referring to vicarious suffering, or suffering for others, as expressed in these words (5): "Surely the suffering servant hath borne our sickness and carried our pains. . . . He was wounded for our transgressions, he was bruised for our iniquities. The chastisement he bore is the health for us, and by his wounds we are healed." This suffering servant did his work in quietness and by the operation of gentle influences. He accepted his role willingly, without complaint, and was compared to sheep, the meekest of animals. This concept of the suffering servant became an integral part of the life of Israel and its people, and also became deeply embedded in the Judeo–Christian tradition. The Prophet Isaiah communicates this message with these words: "By his knowledge shall my righteous servant justify many, for he shall bear their iniquities" (6). The message of the suffering servant refers to the individual, but it can also refer to a community. As community or state, the people of Israel became a collective suffering servant or wounded healer, and have continued to this day to communicate a wounded-but-healing image, as illustrated in these words, ancient but ever new, used to describe Israel: " . . . a light to lighten the Gentiles and for the glory of my people Israel."

In the Asklepian tradition of healing, a paradox is at the heart of the mystery: The healer heals, but at the same time the healer remains wounded. No one is without wounds, to be sure, but the underlying principle of the mystery relates to a knowledge of a wound of which the true healer is forever aware.

The critical question is why does the healer have to have knowledge (awareness) of his or her own wound, and why does he or she need to participate in the wound or share it again and again to effect the cure? Further, does this endeavor of the healer have a relationship to knowledge of, and participation in, the wounds of the patient? These questions can be answered, Groesbeck points out, by understanding the message of the myth of Asklepios as reflected in the transference relationship of doctor and patient (7): "The ill patient seeks an outer healer, but the inner healer or healing factor is also activated. Real cure cannot take place without the action of this inner healing factor" (p. 135). When ill, the patient ought to activate the *inner physician* or *healer*, that is, the inner healing powers, or the curative powers of the self. This may not take place or be integrated into the patient's consciousness, however, if the patient projects his or her own inner healing powers onto the doctor. At the same time, the doctor's inner wounded side is activated by contact with the sick person, and can easily be projected onto the patient rather than contained within the doctor. If the relationship remains one in which both patient and doctor maintain their unconscious projections each upon the other, no real healing occurs. The doctor must be in touch at the deepest level with his or her own wounds, or *inner patient*, so that these wounds are not projected upon the patient. Equally important, the patient must be in touch with the healer within, and not project this inner healer onto the doctor.

In essence, as Groesbeck observes, both participants must experience the health–sickness polarity if the patient is to be freed and healed (8). Healing is interfered with when the doctor identifies only with the healer polarity and projects his or her inner wounds and illnesses onto the patient, or when the patient is estranged from his or her inner healer, projecting it onto the doctor. The true healer does not stand outside of the healing experience as a disinterested observer but must be ready to have his or her own wounds activated and reactivated (contained within and not projected). In a sense, the true healer remains forever a patient as well as a healer, and works with that deep and abiding awareness. In such a healing encounter, the patient finds more than a cure of symptoms, but discovers the meaning of his or her illness through a genuine understanding of his or her part in the illness and the healing experience.

Other factors may be mentioned in describing the encounter between the wounded healer and the patient. The healer takes wounds of mortality, vulnerability, and pain into the encounter and is able to remain in the presence of dying, suffering patients who show the healer the intimacy of their hurts. The wounded healer is thus seen, in this context, not just as a helper but as one who can be helped. The wounded healer enters the encounter as one who not only can give but who also can receive. Often the highest form of giving is receiving, a letting in, a letting it happen. When patients sense that they can give something, that they can be helpful, the scene changes—from people there to be helped, to people there to be helpful. Patients want to get well, but they do not want to be forced into being dependent on doctors who are active, controlling agents. Patients themselves want to be active participants in the healing endeavor.

. Possibly the greatest message in the wounded-healer concept is that those in the healing and helping professions see themselves not only as helpers but also as persons who need to be helped. They then enter the healing encounter with an openness to receive. This openness, this sensitivity, even an awareness of brokenness and mortality, set the stage for healing to flow back and forth between patient and healer. One cannot enter this healing arena as a healer, however, unless one's wounds are recognized and accepted. Does not the Biblical adage, "physician, heal thyself," tell us this? Does it not tell us that the doctor is not separated form the patient, for the doctor, too, is in search of healing. In a sense, the doctor in *Macbeth* is echoing this same message when he says, "Therein the patient must minister to himself." Thus, professionalism takes on a false sense when it becomes a barrier between patient and doctor and interferes with what Martin Buber has described as the I–Thou encounter, a subject-to-subject meeting. The true healer's involvement is I–Thou and not I–It, subject-to-object, the relationship that Buber calls the curse of our day (9). Only in the I–Thou relationship can the patient see and experience the wounds of the healer and find that life and death are found in the same figure.

Henri Nouwen, in his book, *The Wounded Healer*, reminds us of an old Talmudic legend that communicates a profound message for healing (10). The story is of a rabbi who asked the Prophet Elijah when the Messiah would come. Elijah replied that the rabbi should ask the Messiah directly and that he would find him sitting at the gates of the city. "How will I know him?" the rabbi asked. Elijah replied, "He is sitting among the poor covered with wounds. The others unbind all their wounds at the same time and then bind them up again. But he unbinds one at a time and binds it up again saying to himself, 'Perhaps I shall be needed. If so, I must always be ready so as not to delay for a moment.'" He recognized his wounds, let them show, and made them available as a source of healing.

As Nouwen points out, the theme of the wounded healer implies that all grace, growth, and healing are communicated or incited by starting with the humanity, brokenness, and vulnerability of both the healer and the person to be healed. These, in both, must be affirmed. The aim of the true healer is not so much to remove the pain of life as to interpret it. The evidence in the healer of woundedness or pain and of the transcendence or constructive endurance of it help to heal the patient.

Let us now turn to illustrations taken both from life and literature to see how the healing power of wounds is found, not only in the consulting rooms of doctors and clergy, but also in those who share their wounds in their work or in their written or spoken words.

Members of Alcoholics Anonymous (AA) fit well the category of wounded healers. These persons have had their lives laid bare and pushed to the brink of destruction by alcoholism and its accompanying problems. When these persons arise from the ashes of the hellfire of addictive bondage, they have an understanding, sensitivity, and willingness to enter into and maintain healing encounters with their fellow alcoholics. In this encounter, they cannot and will not permit themselves to forget their brokenness and vulnerability. Their wounds are acknowledged, accepted, and kept visible. Further, their wounds are used to illuminate and stabilize their own lives while they work to bring the healing of sobriety to their alcoholic brothers and sisters, and sometimes to their sons and daughters. The effectiveness of AA's members in the care and treatment of their fellow alcoholics is one of the great success stories of our time, and graphically illustrates the power of wounds, when used creatively, to lighten the burden of pain and suffering.

Ernest Hemingway understood well the creative healing power in one's wounds and urged his troubled fellow writer, F. Scott Fitzgerald, to finish *Tender Is the Night*: "Forget your personal tragedy. We are all bitched from the start and you especially have to hurt like hell before you can write seriously. But when you get the damned hurt use it—don't cheat with it. Be as faithful to it as a scientist. . . . " (11, p. 408). William Butler Yeats wrote out of his wounds, for as Auden said of him "mad Ireland hurt him into poetry." Rainer Maria Rilke, in his *Letters to a Young Poet*, wrote in reference to himself (12): "Do not believe that he who seeks to comfort you lives untroubled among the simple and quiet words that sometimes do you good. His life has much difficulty and sadness and remains far behind yours. Were it otherwise he would never have been able to find these words" (p. 72). Rilke is saying that his words of comfort and healing flow from his own wounds or sadness and life's difficulties. His wounds of pain and sadness had awakened his imagination, his creativity, his care of people.

The renowned Spanish writer, theologian, and existential philosopher, Miguel de Unamuno, writes of a priest, living in a small Spanish village, who is loved by all the people for his piety, his kindness, and the majesty with which he celebrates the Mass. To his people, he is already a saint, and they speak of him as Saint Don Emmanuel. He helps them with their plowing and planting, tends them when they are sick, hears their confessions, comforts them in death, and every Sunday, in his rich, lilting voice, lifts them to the gates of heaven with his chanting. Actually, Don Emmanuel is not so much a saint as he is a martyr. Long ago his own faith left him. He is an atheist, a good man doomed to endure the life of a hypocrite, pretending to a faith he does not really have. As he raises the chalice of wine, his hands tremble, a cold sweat pours from his brow, but he cannot stop, for he knows that the people need this of him, and that their need is greater than his sacrifice. Could it be that Don Emmanuel's whole life is a kind of prayer, a song of joy to God (13)? He preserved hope in those whom he served, when there was no hope within himself (14). He helped God become alive in all he touched.

Who is this Unamuno, who wrote of Don Emmanuel? Figuratively, Unamuno, in writing about Don Emmanuel, is writing about himself. He viewed life as a ceaseless struggle between reason and faith, and saw his philosophic role as that of consoling humankind, of making life easier to live. His own terror of extinction became a wound that enhanced his power to heal and enabled grace and hope to enter his own life. In spite of success and recognition, his wounds remained with him, including an exile from his homeland and condemnation for heresy. Doubt and uncertainty gripped him, and he lived with the agonizing affirmation, "I believe, helpest Thou my unbelief." His writings are made unique by the central theme of his own spiritual search for the meaning of life and death. Revealing his own vulnerabilities and ambiguities, he holds everyone who listens. Readers, traveling with Unamuno through the dark night of the soul, are drawn into his writings and become their own interpreters. Unamuno asked that, if characters of a story are the product of an author's dream, may not human beings be God's dream? To continue to exist he saw as the human's profoundest prayer. Thus, he prayed (15): "Dream us, O Lord."

Similar to Unamuno, Leo Tolstoy in his writings unwrapped his own wounds while dressing those of his readers. In the end, both found healing. Tolstoy's wound was his fear of death and his struggle to accept his own mortality, the awful truth that he too one day would die. Through his fear he taught us to work through our own feelings about death. In his short story, *The Death of Ivan Ilyich*, one of the most powerful of literary works on the subject of death and dying, he mirrors his own struggle and his own triumph. Writing 100 years before the work of Kubler-Ross, he describes the same stages of the dying process and criticizes the same attitudes toward death that Kubler-Ross condemns in her seminal work (17, 18). Through his wound, persisting at some level to his final days, he has lighted with new meanings a path that each of us must travel.

A beautiful example of the wounded healer is described in Thornton Wilder's *The Angel That Troubled the Waters*, a one-act play based on the biblical story, in John 5:1-4, of how the Pool of Bethesda could heal whenever an angel troubled its waters (19). In this play, a physician comes periodically to the Pool of Bethesda and waits for the angel, hoping to be the first in the pool and to be healed of his melancholy and remorse. The angel appears, but blocks the physician just as he is ready to step into the water and be healed. The angel tells the physician to draw back, for this moment is not for him. The physician pleads with the angel, but the angel insists that healing is not for him. The physician pleads with the angel, but the angel insists that healing is not for him. The dialogue continues between the physician and the angel—and then these telling words from the angel: "Without your wound where would your power be? It is your melancholy that makes your low voice tremble into the hearts of men. The very angels themselves cannot persuade the wretched and blundering children on earth as can one human being broken on the wheels of living. In Love's service only the wounded soldiers can serve. Draw back" (p. 149).

Later, the person who was healed rejoiced in his good fortune and turned to the physician before leaving the Pool of Bethesda and said: "But come with me first, an hour only, to my home. My son is lost in dark thoughts. I—I do not understand him, and only you have ever lifted his mood. Only an hour. . . . My daughter, since her child has died, sits in the shadow. She will not listen to us . . . but she will listen to you" (p. 149).

And now an example of an old truth discovered anew in the New World. In late 1528, a handful of Spaniards, survivors of an ill-starred expedition to Florida, were washed ashore in the Gulf of Mexico, probably near the present site of Galveston, Texas. One of these men was Alvar Nunez Cabeza de Vaca, 38 years old, the lieutenant of the expedition, an adaptable man with a reserve of great inner strength and renewal. Despite the privations he had endured, Cabeza de Vaca led two other Spaniards and a Moor on a journey across the entire continent, barefoot and often naked, that took them eight years.

De Vaca eventually managed to get back to Spain by way of Mexico City and sent a report in the form of a letter to his king, relating what had befallen him. The letter begins as the usual story of a European adventurer who leaves home to exploit people. Little by little, De Vaca finds out, however, that people are his brothers and sisters, and feels genuine concern for them. He seems afraid that his king might not be interested in what he has to say, for it is the story of a disaster in Spanish colonial history and in the king's personal finances. In the world of the individual, nonetheless, it is a story of triumph.

The Indians demanded that de Vaca and his companions cure their sick. When the Spaniards said they did not know how, the Indians withheld food from them and threatened to kill them. Thus they had to heal the Indians or die. They prayed for strength and developed techniques of breathing on the patients, making the sign of the cross, and reciting certain prayers. The patients began to get well, and de Vaca and his companions were astounded at their power to heal. The sick came from everywhere, it seemed. De Vaca and his companions kept their powers to heal throughout their journey across this continent. It has been said that de Vaca found the limitless within the narrowly limited. He helped when he had no means of helping, and he gave when he had nothing to give (20–22).

When de Vaca finally returned to Spain he noticed that his interest in healing, and to some extent his power to heal, had slipped away amid his affluence and the affluence of his home country. He wrote to his king:

> While with them I thought only about doing the Indians good. But back among my fellow countrymen, I had to be on guard not to lose such a concern. If one lives where all suffer and starve, one acts on one's own impulse to help. But where plenty abounds, we surrender

our generosity, believing that our country replaces us each and several. This is not so, and is indeed a delusion. On the contrary, the power of maintaining life in others lives within each of us, and from each of us does it recede when unused. It is a concentrated power. If you are not acquainted with it, your Majesty can have no inkling of what it is like, what it portends, or the ways in which it slips from one. Your majesty, by your grace, farewell (20, pp. 36–37).

G. Adler, writing insightfully about wounds and healing, describes well de Vaca's discovery as he explored the new world of America (23): "To be wounded means also to have the healing power activated in us; or might we possibly say that without being wounded one would never meet just this healing power?" (p. 18).

Closer home, in our journey with wounded healers, we cannot overlook Sigmund Freud or Carl Jung. Their wounds were many. With these wounds they have helped to heal us and themselves. Their lives and work are too well known for any more than a brief comment here, but a review will reveal a tapestry of tragedy and triumph.

Think of Vienna's anti-Semitic atmosphere, which surrounded Freud's life; Freud's struggles with religion; his loss of his symbolic son, Jung; his cancer of the jaw; his confrontation with the Nazis; and his exile from his homeland. Think of Jung, and the impact of what may have been a psychotic breakdown; his struggles with the dark side of God; the rupture with his symbolic father, Freud; and the accusation of his being a Nazi sympathizer. These are only a few of the many incidents in the lives of Freud and Jung that made them wounded pilgrims.

Think of psychiatrist Harry Stack Sullivan, an isolated and lonely man, who knew mental illness through personal experience. At the Sheppard and Enoch Pratt Hospital in Maryland he found himself truly at home in treating "untreatable" schizophrenic patients. Imprinted by wounds of loneliness, Sullivan sensed that the lonely ones on the psychiatric wards, the withdrawn psychotic patients, were suffering from an illness the inner surface of which he knew. Could these patients be suffering from a deficiency disease, that is, the lack of intimacy? Because he knew both loneliness and intimacy, a healing relationship was created with his patients, in which intimacy became that situation involving two people that permits validation of all components of personal worth (24, 25). With too many wounds for self-satisfaction and with too much pride to conceal these wounds, he was seen by patients and colleagues as truly a wounded healer, who knew personally the meaning of the stark Biblical words, "Physician, heal thyself." Healing for Sullivan did not depend on the doctor's cleverness at deciphering the secret code of the patient but on the doctor's and patient's shared humanness and mutual respect for the ambiguity and complexity inherent in human existence.

One of our contemporaries who carries his words, both written and spoken, across our land, stands as an apt model of the wounded healer. Surgeon Richard Selzer is an excellent modern example of the wounded healer, as illustrated by much of his writings. Selzer's wound is the wound of empathy with the patient. Selzer takes on the patient's brokenness and lack of wholeness, and when the patient is healed, Selzer receives the grace of healing for himself. Selzer recognizes that, in genuine healing, the doctor is also involved in treating the doctor. So the doctor's ceaseless efforts when all is hopeless should never be denigrated. Selzer describes the doctor–patient encounter (26): "A doctor gazes at the patient and sees himself; joined they are one pilgrim in search of health" (pp. 63–64). Selzer speaks of an operation as an enactment of the biblical story of Jonah and the whale. In the surgical procedure, the patient as whale swallows up the surgeon as Jonah. Unlike Jonah, the surgeon does not resist the journey but willingly descends into the sick body in order to cut out of it the part that threatens to kill it. In an operation where the patient is healed, the surgeon is spewed out of the whale's body, and both surgeon and patient are healed. In an operation where the patient dies on the operating table, the surgeon, although rescued from the whale and the sea of blood, is not fully healed but will bear forever after the scars of the sojourn in the patient's belly (27).

Among our great forebears in the clergy, we find that their secret in changing the world, themselves, and others was anchored in a wound imprinted on body and soul. When John Wesley—

Oxford professor, preacher, and founder of the Methodist Church —was five years old, he was the last member of his large family rescued when their home burned down. Wesley, appearing at an upstairs window with the flames raging around him, was pulled from the burning house by a neighbor standing on the shoulders of another. This experience made a deep and lasting impression on him, for he often referred to himself as a brand plucked from the burning by God. Like Asklepios in the Greek myth, he was snatched from the fires. His life covered almost the entire eighteenth century, and the imprint of death upon his life was carried as an energizing wound, as he wrote hundreds of articles and books, working with thousands of people from the slums of London to the Oglethorpe Colony in Georgia. As an organizer and agent for change in the personal lives of people, there were few who could equal him. In his ministry, dogma was never a separating factor, for he transcended that with the subject-to-subject or I-thou encounter, expressed always in these words: "If your heart is as my heart give me your hand." Throughout his tumultuous life he was a healer with wounds. He never saw himself beyond the need for healing. He searched for and found the healing encounter (28).

Harry Emerson Fosdick of Riverside Church fame in New York City had a depressive breakdown during his student days at Union Theological Seminary and was hospitalized for several months. The experience opened to him a lifetime of vulnerability and empathy. As preacher and pastor, his counselling ministry led him into an approach to preaching in which his sermons became personal counselling on a group scale. People from everywhere flocked to Riverside to be a part of his care. As he counselled parishioners who enumerated their almost unbearable symptoms, he often stopped them, saying, "Don't you tell me, let me tell you how you feel." When he finished, wide-eyed parishioners often exclaimed, "My Lord! How did you know that?" He knew because he had been there, and was also now there with them. He was no stranger to their neurotic agony with its waves of melancholia, obsessive anxieties, and suicidal ruminations. Without his wounds, would there have been such power of healing in his pulpit or in his pastoral counselling (29)?

Anton T. Boisen, theologian and father of the clinical pastoral training movement, has described his descent into the depths of psychotic illness and his arduous journey back to health (30). His firm conviction, demonstrated by his own experience, that mental illness could be an opportunity for greater understanding of self and the human condition has inspired and informed those concerned with the problems of the emotionally disturbed. During his college days, following a lonely childhood, he had difficulty establishing personal relationships. At first he turned to the rugged outdoor life of the Forest Service, then he trained in the seminary for the ministry, and during World War I he worked overseas with the YMCA. None of these endeavors seemed to bring him fulfillment. Later, his work as a young pastor also proved unhappy. No venture seemed to solve his inner problems. Then a serious mental breakdown overwhelmed him. While suffering severe stress, Boisen had a valid religious experience which was accompanied by or followed quickly by a psychosis. Resemblances between the onset of acute schizophrenia and religious experience not infrequently can be seen, and no one has spoken of this more vividly than Boisen. Buffeted into retreat from the world, he underwent a genuine spiritual rebirth. When he reestablished his bonds to the real world, he brought with him a message which moved his contemporaries to the depths. His unswerving belief that emotional illness could have positive use led him to become one of the first chaplains in a psychiatric hospital; to father clinical pastoral training in seminaries; and, through research, teaching, writing, and patient care, to make an authentic and monumental contribution to the psychology of religion. His friend, Harry Stack Sullivan, spoke of Boisen's wounds and healing power as flowing from his courage, his depth and tenderness of feeling, and his clear insight into his own brokenness and that of those to whom he ministered.

Healing comes through the wounded life. True healers, by virtue of coping with their own suffering and in remaining fully aware of their own vulnerabilities, become pilgrims with others on the path to healing. They demonstrate anew in their work the profound linkages between the wounded healer of medicine and the suffering servant of the Judeo–Christian tradition.

References

1. Guggenbuhl-Craig A: Power in the Helping Professions. New York, Spring Publications, 1971

2. Jung CG: Fundamental questions of psychotherapy. Collected Works 16:116, 1951

3. Kerenyi C: Asklepios: Archetypal Image of the Physician's Existence. Translated by Manheim R. New York, Pantheon Books, 1959

4. Meier CA: Ancient Incubation and Modern Psychotherapy. Translated by Curtis M. Evanston IL, Northwestern University Press, 1967

5. Isaiah 53:4–5

6. Isaiah 53:11

7. Groesbeck CJ, Taylor B: The psychiatrist as wounded physician. Am J Psychoanal 37:131–139, 1977

8. Groesbeck CJ: The archetypal image of the wounded healer. J Anal Psychol 20:122–145, 1975

9. Buber M: I–Thou. New York, Scribners, 1970

10. Nouwen HJM: The Wounded Healer: Ministry in Contemporary Society. New York, Doubleday, 1972

11. Baker C: Ernest Hemingway: Selected Letters, 1917–1961. New York, Scribners, 1981

12. Rilke RM: Letters to a Young Poet. Translated by Norton MDH. New York, WW Norton, 1962

13. Selzer R: Mortal Lessons: Notes on the Art of Surgery. New York, Simon and Schuster, 1976

14. Unamuno M de: Abel Sanchez and Other Stories. Translated by Kerrigan A. Chicago, Regnery, 1956

15. Tibbetts OL: Renewing acquaintance with Unamuno. Christian Century 98:585–586 May 20, 1981

16. Tolstoy L: The Death of Ivan Ilyich and Selected Tales. Washington DC, National Home Library Foundation, 1935

17. Soudek IH: Waiting for the end: a study of the similarities between Elizabeth Kubler-Ross's On Death and Dying and Leo Tolstoy's The Death of Ivan Ilyich. Pharos 43:9, 1979

18. Kubler-Ross E: On Death and Dying. New York, Macmillan, 1969

19. Wilder TN: The Angel That Troubled the Waters and Other Plays. New York, Coward-McCann, 1928

20. Long H: The Power Within Us: Cabeza de Vaca's Relation of His Journey from Florida to the Pacific, 1528–1536. New York, Duell, Sloan, and Pearce [no date]

21. Nunez Cabeza de Vaca A: Adventures in the Unknown Interior of America. Translated and annotated by Cavey C. Albuquerque, University of New Mexico Press, 1983

22. Lewis BR: North American El Dorado. American History Illustrated 17:11–19, 1982

23. Adler G: Notes regarding the dynamics of the self, in Dynamic Aspects of the Psyche. New York, Analytical Psychology Club, 1956

24. Perry HS: Psychiatrist of America: The Life of Harry Stack Sullivan. Cambridge MA, Belknap Press, 1982

25. Brady D: Review of HS Perry's Psychiatrist of America: The Life of Harry Stack Sullivan. J Am Acad Psychoanal 12:289–292, 1984

26. Selzer R: Confessions of a Knife. New York, Simon and Schuster, 1979

27. Selzer R: Letters to a Young Doctor. New York, Simon and Schuster, 1982

28. Heitzenrater RP: The Elusive Mr. Wesley. Nashville, Abingdon Press, 1984

29. Fosdick HE: The Living of These Days: The Autobiography of Harry Emerson Fosdick. New York, Harper, 1956

30. Boisen AT: Out of the Depths—An Autobiographical Study of Mental Disorder and Religious Experience. New York, Harper, 1960

4

Minister and Healer: Each as the Other

James A. Knight, M.D., B.D., M.P.H.

4

Minister and Healer:
Each as the Other

Although *healing* and *ministry*, as well as *healer* and *minister*, are
words with strong linkages in our language, we seldom pay proper
honor to their deep and abiding relationship.

The term ministry comes from the Latin word for service.
Thus, minister is defined as servant—one who waits upon or
ministers to the needs of another. As the New Testament word for
servant (*diakonos*), it has its origin in Jesus' work, expressed in the
statement: "The Son of man came not to be ministered unto but to
minister" (1). The relationship of servant and minister is further
emphasized in the New Testament admonition that "whosoever
will be great among you, let him be your minister, and whosoever
will be chief among you, let him be your servant" (2).

The healing dimension of ministry becomes clear when we
recognize that the *soter*, the saviour (precisely, the *healer*), means
to make healthy and whole. The mythological symbol of saviour
or healer (which was applied to the man Jesus) shows most clearly
the unity of the religious and the medical (3). When salvation is
understood in the sense of healing, the most intimate relation can
be seen between the religious and the medical, and the terms *minister as healer* and *healer as minister* become meaningful in their
fullest sense. Further, the relationship between minister and healer
can be expressed as each-within-the-other or each as the other.

Although the facets of ministry are many and varied (4), the minister as the bearer of salvation or health has seldom been better described than in Thomas Fuller's tribute to William Perkins in 1642: "An excellent surgeon at the jointing of a broken soul and at easing a doubtful conscience" (5, p. ix).

In speaking of the minister as healer and healer as minister, one is emphasizing that the ministry of each is a healing vocation. This healing vocation may encompass, but extends far beyond, scientific technology to include a quality of mystery—the *gift* of healing. This quality is tied to charismatic authority.

To comprehend the full dimension of charismatic authority, one should reflect on the definition of charisma: spiritual power and virtue attributed to a person who is regarded as set apart from the ordinary—set apart by reason of a special relation to that which is considered of ultimate value.

The minister and the doctor are the two professionals who have managed to keep their charismatic authority, although other professionals have sought it and perhaps held it briefly in history. They both have an ancient link with charismatic authority represented by the biblical "power to heal sickness and to cast out demons" (6). Many in our society fear that, as minister and doctor become more closely associated with governmental agencies and institutions, they will become civil servants and lose their charismatic authority. In other words, the minister and doctor will endure not as mediators of the mysteries of life and death, but as civil-service technicians in the health enterprise.

Such a prediction is partly nonsense, because of the priestly dimension of both the minister's and the doctor's roles. In our culture, especially in matters of health, charismatic authority has to do with the possibility of death in any illness, which accounts for the seriousness of the healing endeavor. Also, too many unknown or unknowable factors exist in illness to depend entirely on technical skill for the restoration of wholeness. In healing, technical skill is accompanied by factors not easily assessed, such as timing, quality, blending, intuitive insights, and exquisite awareness of the right moment for intervention. Thus, healing deals with powerful and mysterious forces that are not completely amenable to reason. In the healing endeavor, then, ministers function in their priestly role; doctors also retain a great deal of their original priestly role.

The human condition which led to charismatic authority is still with us. Because of the frailty of mortal flesh, we ascribe to the minister, as well as to the doctor, a special, more-than-human authority, in the hope that he or she will intervene successfully on our behalf should we fall ill.

No matter what changes occur in healing strategies in society, ministers and doctors need not fear the loss of charismatic authority, as long as they hold to the source of their authority: the conscientious concern for the well-being of those for whom they care; a receptivity to their silent plea, "Don't let me die!"; and the unbroken promise that they will wage an unrelenting battle against death or crippling in the patient's behalf. With such a commitment, one's charismatic authority cannot be interfered with, but will be validated and renewed daily throughout one's life.

To show healing and ministry as strongly linked, it seems appropriate to highlight the minister as healer and the healer as minister.

MINISTER AS HEALER

A major task of the minister is that of healer, and with the healing task come some special opportunities. These special opportunities relate to the therapy of the word, to awakening in all an awareness of the tragic sense of life, to distinguishing between healing and curing, and to the balancing of technology with humanity.

The Therapy of the Word

Such terms as the *therapy of the word* and the *alchemy of the word* are rich in meaning and also lead us to ask about the "word" in the biblical tradition. Proverbs states the issue clearly: "The tongue that brings healing is a tree of life." And Socrates declared, "I would rather write on the hearts of living persons than the skins of dead sheep." The minister as healer cannot be understood fully apart from the therapy of the word.

French poet Arthur Rimbaud (1854–1891) has given us the powerful term, alchemy of the word. Rimbaud saw language as a sacred value, a set of magical spells, aimed at changing life. He spoke of transcending Christianity through more charity and through acceptance of the body, as well as the soul, as vessels of the new truth (7).

In Unamuno's story of the priest Don Emmanuel, the alchemy of the word is beautifully illustrated through Blasillo, the "village idiot." Although many in the village laughed at Blasillo, the priest befriended him and taught him a number of things in spite of Blasillo's mental retardation. In return, Blasillo became close to the priest and was always available to help the priest in a variety of tasks around the church and with the parishioners. In the pageantry of the Good Friday church service, Don Emmanuel moved his parishioners beyond comprehension with these words: "My God, my God, why hast thou forsaken me!" During the following few days Blasillo went about the village quoting those words with the same poignancy and pathos that the priest's voice had carried. Tears came to the eyes of those who heard Blasillo, and people fell to their knees. As Blasillo spoke those words, redemptive healing claimed the people. From feeble lips and a limited mind came the message, and through the alchemy of the word, the broken ones were made whole (8).

In a recent address, Dr. Daniel C. Tosteson, Dean of the Harvard Medical School, stated that as technology in medicine becomes more refined, the character of the tongue [word] of those who care for the sick will play a greater role in healing (9).

The Persians distinguished the *word-doctor* from the *herb-doctor* and the *knife-doctor*. About the word-doctor the Persians said, "This one is the best of all healers who deal with the Holy Word, and he will best drive away sickness from the body of the faithful" (10, p. 186).

In a scholarly book, *The Therapy of the Word in Classical Antiquity*, Dr. Pedro Lain Entralgo traces the gradual refinement of Greek ideas concerning the use of the word for therapy (11).

Early attempts at logotherapy included not only the incantations of magic but also the more acceptable "cheering speech" of Homer. In the Homeric epics, one can collect data on the use of the word for curative purposes. A careful reading of the *Iliad* and the *Odyssey* reveals that the uttering of words on the occasion of human illness takes three forms, each different from the others: the prayer, the magic charm, and the suggestive, cheering speech. It is not surprising, then, that some conceived the idea of applying the persuasive word "technically" to the curing of certain maladies.

Plato states that the suggestive or persuasive word can be called a charm whenever it is a beautiful speech (*logos kalos*) and when, as a result of being such, it produces in the soul *sophrosyne*—a beautiful, harmonious, and rightful ordering of all the ingredients of the psychic life (beliefs, feelings, impulses, knowledge, thoughts, and value judgments). How is this achieved? By organizing the contents of the soul around the axis of its beliefs or by eliciting in it new beliefs and persuasions more noble than the old (11). Plato designates this reorganizing and enlightening process of the persuasive word *katharsis*. Sophrosyne, the harmonious and rightful ordering of all the ingredients of the psychic life, is of importance in healing from a twofold point of view: It produces beneficial somatic effects, and it is a contingent condition for the efficacy of medications. Accordingly, their knowledge would not be "technically" complete, if doctors were unable to produce this harmony and integration in the souls of their patients. The therapy of the word thereby acquires intellectual justification in the healing of the sick.

The therapeutic power of the word was understood by physicians, philosophers, priests, poets, and dramatists of ancient Greece, from Homer through Hippocrates, Plato, and Aristotle. Yet a dominant trait of our healing strategies has been their strongly somatic orientation. Western medicine, throughout most of its history, has disregarded the power of the word in the treatment of human illness, and placed its faith in treatments such as surgical procedures, drugs, and diets.

This dominant trait in Western medicine had its origin in the naturalistic medicine of classical Greece, roughly speaking in the fifth century B.C. Healers in preclassical Greece employed (alone, or in combination with other forms of treatment) the therapeutic power of the word. The outlines of Greek natural science became discernible, and in the fifth century B.C. Hippocratic medicine appeared. To achieve its scientific naturalism, Hippocratic medicine had first to reject the old verbal therapy. Medicine or healing for the Hippocratic physicians became the "mute art," as Virgil was later to call it. Acts, not words, were used to treat illness. Hippocratic physicians were concerned with the nature of the body (*soma*), and not with divine or daemonic powers or with the soul of the patient.

The question has been asked, "Was a flaw already discernible in the well-laid foundations of Greek medicine as early as the fifth century B.C.?" Probably so, for in the *Charmides* of Plato the physicians of Greece are said to be wanting in an appreciation of the significance of the whole and deficient in the treatment of those ailments of the body brought on by the soul (12). A young man, Charmides (in that dialogue), complains about a headache. He wants a particular drug, but Socrates explains to him at length that this simple treatment is not adequate. "To treat the head by itself, apart from the body as a whole," he says, "is utter folly" (p. 206). The ideal approach had been described to him (Socrates) by a Thracian physician:

You ought not to attempt to cure eyes
Without head,
Or head without body,
So you should not treat body
Without soul.

As Lain Entralgo shows quite clearly, Hippocratic physicians were acquainted with the far-reaching changes in the body that might be produced by emotional disturbances. At the same time, because they were aware of the emotional factors, they used treatments that were somatic (11). Although they knew that words could and should be used on occasion to suggest, cheer, exhort, or persuade, they had no technique of verbal therapy.

In general, it can be stated that Western physicians recognized clearly that disturbances of the mind or soul could and did cause many kinds of bodily disturbances, alone or in combination with other factors. Yet they held that their business was to treat the body, and that the mind or soul was not within their province. Thus, for centuries, the canon of medical studies that became established in the universities of Europe was essentially that laid down by Galen, who relied mainly on Hippocratic sources. Until the introduction of psychiatry into the medical curriculum within the past century, it remained in principle unchanged.

The Tragic Sense of Life.

This task relates to awakening in all the tragic sense of life, to awareness of the inevitability of death. To better understand this task, one can again learn something from the way of the ancient Greeks. In their sense of the tragic, the Greeks did show human-kind that pain could exalt and, in tragedy, for a moment people could have sight of a meaning usually beyond their grasp. Euripides makes the old Trojan queen say, in her extremity: "Yet had God not turned us in his hand and cast to earth our greatness, we would have passed away giving nothing to men. They would have found no theme for song in us nor made great poems from our sorrows" (13, p. 171).

Edith Hamilton, in *The Greek Way to Western Civilization*, states that in Greek tragedy the figures are seen simply, from afar, parts of a whole having no beginning and no end, and yet their remoteness does not diminish their profoundly tragic and individual appeal (13). She goes on to say that there is a more familiar masterpiece that can help one understand this method, the life of Christ, a tragedy after the Greek model. The figure of Christ is outlined with simplicity, and yet he could not be thought of as a type. The Gospel writers never let one know what went on within when the words they record were spoken and the deeds they tell of were done. For example, "And Peter said, man, I know not what thou sayest. And immediately, while he yet spoke, the cock crowed. And the Lord turned, and looked upon Peter" (Luke 22:61-62).

The sense of the tragic is described by Hamilton in these moving words:

> Our sense of the tragedy of the Gospels does not come from our identifying ourselves with Christ nor from any sense of deep personal knowledge. He is given to us more simply drawn than any other character anywhere, and more unmistakable in His individuality than any other. He stands upon the tremendous stage of the conflict of good and evil for mankind, and we are far removed; we can only watch. That agony is of another sort from ours. Yet never, by no other spectacle, has the human heart been so moved to pity and awe. And after some such fashion the Greek dramatists worked (4, p. 241).

Something here relates to the minister as healer, who in healing does embrace the tragic sense of life, who in each human being sees humanity, who in each person sees an individual but one connected with something universal. Thus, with feeling, acceptance, and suffering, a special dimension is brought to the life of the patient. Possibly Nietzsche had this dimension in mind when he spoke of the "reaffirmation of the will to live in the face of death and the joy of its inexhaustibility when so reaffirmed."

Healing as More Than Curing

To be effective in their work, ministers as healers must not lose sight of a distinction their priestly forebears made between curing and healing. This distinction was certainly recognized in ancient Greece, especially at the Temple of Asklepios (14), where curing involved removing the cause of disease. Healing involved something more, for it was a treatment of the whole person, not merely the symptoms. Thus, it involved psychological, religious, physical, and social factors, and the patient could go out from the temple feeling restored in health. Supervising the process created in the healer or priest a deep sense of humility. Humility was a part of the priestly tradition, appropriate to one who was an intermediary between the person and God. The healer was only an instrument—one who could promise neither cure nor healing (15).

Balancing Technology With Humanity

The minister as healer can help all involved in healing understand why too much technology and too little humanity have been a recurring theme in the criticism of medicine and of the healing strategies for most of the last two centuries. Machines have separated doctor from patient, and the closeness to and touching by the doctor have been replaced by electrodes, wires, tubes, scopes, and monitors. The doctor tends the machine that tends the patient, and the healing power of the hands that touch and comfort are lost through our awesome but often dehumanizing technology. What happened that our healing endeavors became so scientific and we lost so easily the true art of healing?

Two philosophical positions, themselves derived from historical forces in Western culture, may explain how discrepant attitudes toward medicine and doctors have come about: a) mind–body dualism, the doctrine that separates the psychological and the somatic, and b) reductionism, the view that complex phenomena are ultimately derivative from a single primary principle (16). These two philosophical attitudes have been decisive in determining that scientific medicine in the West has concentrated on the body and not on the mind, and that disease has become conceptualized in somatic and not in psychological or social terms. They have fostered the notion of the body as a machine; of disease, as the consequence of breakdown of the machine; and the doctor's task, as repair of the machine. This view is essentially today's biomedical model, which holds that disease ultimately can be reduced to physiochemical events, and treatment to correction of underlying biochemical derangements.

The emphasis all along has been more on the technological challenges of treating disease than on the consideration of the religious, psychological, and social dimensions of illness and patienthood. Within the biomedical establishment, the applicability of the scientific method to the study of psychosocial processes is viewed with skepticism. The psychosocial is relegated to the category of art and is deemed neither approachable by scientific study nor capable of being taught or learned (16).

Much needs to be done to convince students of the healing arts that the outcome of their interventions with patients may depend less on their technical skills than on the quality of their relationships with patients, and their knowledge of the patient's life situation. In other words, much needs to be done to convince those in healing that the real task is more the laying on of hands and less the reading of complex signals from machines (17, 18). Relevant to this task is the counsel of the renowned physician Sir William Osler: "It is more important to know what sort of patient has a disease than what sort of disease a patient has."

THE HEALER AS MINISTER

The healer-as-minister concept ties us to the distant past when the healing and priestly roles were combined in the same person. Although we are far removed from that ancient heritage, residues of it persist in our healing endeavors and in the perception of our work. Terms still meaningful today come to mind, such as *Vocatio Dei* and *priesthood of all believers*. We see a divine perspective in our work, with religious awe and reverence undergirding it. Many physicians' oaths and covenants acknowledge this spiritual dimension, such as the oath taken by the graduates of the relatively new medical school in the troubled city of Jerusalem: " . . . and we shall seek to fathom the soul of the sick, to restore their spirit, through understanding and compassion."

Priesthood of All Believers and *Vocatio Dei*

In the concept of healer as minister, the implication is that one functions in this role as a special kind of servant. In healing, one is truly a minister, one is set apart because the task is more than human.

At the same time, such a role is distinctly a part of the biblical concept of the priesthood of all believers—what certain medieval preachers and mystics characterized by the impressive term *Voca-*

tio Dei, "divine calling," declaring that certain experiences cannot be called secular and others religious, but that religion can and should pervade all of life. The *Vocatio Dei* is a calling forth of all of one's capacities and skills into worship and work for the common good, a calling by a power greater than oneself or the world in which one lives. The *Vocatio Dei* is a reassertion of the ancient premise that worship and work belong together, that the adoration of God should be integral to everyday life. Thus, the healer's vocation implies a call. Called by whom and to what? The call is from God, and it is a call to life. Whoever we are and whatever we do, we are ministers of God. As David Maitland has said (19): "It is to rescue men, to return them to that life of wholeness in relationship to Himself, that God extends His call of judgment and mercy" (p. 371).

A young woman chaplain, Nina Herrmann, on the staff of a children's hospital, has written of a surgeon at her hospital, in a book entitled *Go out in Joy* (20). While on a European trip, the surgeon met the parents of a young child with a serious brain problem involving a complicated aneurysm. He told the parents that if they brought the child to his hospital in the United States there was a chance he could operate successfully on him. The parents accepted the suggestion, brought their son to this country, and had the surgeon operate.

After the operation, the chaplain met the surgeon as he came out of the operating room, still in his scrub suit. He asked her to walk with him to his office, for he had brought her a small gift from Paris. She tells how, at that moment, she was more fascinated by the doctor's face than with the gift. He had just stood for a good part of 12 hours performing an operation that could make medical history. His face reflected every moment of the fear and exhilaration that had gone into it. She could barely carry on the amenities because she wanted to remember his face. She then went back to her office and wrote of what she had seen. Maybe she overstates what she saw, or describes it too dramatically, but I believe that her words give us a message, a message of what real healing is all about, of what is meant by the healer as minister. These are her words:

... But in the vacuum of moments just after that surgery,
I saw what the journals could not see;
What the textbooks will not record;
What the surgeon himself cannot understand.
For I glimpsed the mystery of what LIFE costs another human being.
I saw in his eyes,
In his face,
In his body,
The terrible price he pays.
And suddenly, for a moment,
I touched the reason for the transcendent mystery of God.
Because, for a moment,
I touched the transcendent mystery of a man's soul. (20, p. 123)

Divine Framework

Healers as ministers bring the scope of their work within a divine framework and perspective. Into the healing relationship God is implied or introduced as a third party. This dimension is expressed succinctly by a well-known maxim that guided psychiatrist Carl Jung's work: *Vocatus atque non vocatus Deus aberit*—Invited, even not invited, God is present.

All Healing Comes From God

Underlying our work is the premise that all healing comes from God, whether God is called by that name or another, such as *nature* or *homeostasis*. It is the recognition and acknowledgement of such a power that leads to the attitude of reverence in our work and in relationship with human life. This recognition gives us a fixed point of reference, a final cause and a final answer, by which to orient our human efforts. Further, there is no hierarchy of healing. Each of us brings to bear professional skills (one's training), one's gift of self (the person as an instrument of healing), and one's organization (for example, the sacramental and group life of the church) in the healing of the sick person. Since all healing comes from God, as persons involved in a healing ministry, we are involved mostly in helping remove the obstacles to healing or strengthening the healing dimension in the patient. Sixteenth-century French surgeon Ambrose Pare described the situation clearly: "God heals the wound; I merely dress it."

Religious Awe and Reverence

If religious awe and reverence undergird the minister's life, then the healer as minister is heir to this heritage. For example, think of the confrontation with the holy that comes about in our care of our patients. One of the most deeply moving religious experiences I have ever had took place in the delivery room of the Duke University Hospital, during my internship. I had delivered a woman of a healthy baby and was waiting for the placenta to separate from the uterus and be expelled by it. Everything had gone well with both mother and infant. One could now see and hear the trickle of blood from the uterus, indicating the placental separation. Shortly thereafter the placenta was expelled and the uterus contracted to shut off the flow of blood. While marvelling at the mystery and miracle of each step in the birth process, I looked out of the window and saw the rays of the early morning sun illuminating the tower of the Duke University Chapel. A most profound sense of the awareness and presence of the holy overwhelmed me. My mind's ear seemed to hear a voice: "Put off your shoes from your feet, for the place on which you are standing is holy ground."

Acceptance and Divine Forgiveness

The healer as minister recognizes that all kinds of moral issues emerge during treatment and healing. We participate in healing with what we ourselves are, as well as with our studied arts. No science dealing with humans can be divorced from problems of philosophy and ethics. Within the structure of human personality and of society, moral values have a reality of their own. These moral values are as real as sexual drives, aggression, and love.

A task that looms large for the healer as minister is the priestly work of bringing acceptance and divine forgiveness to those who may be described as having "overburdened consciences and despairing souls." In other words, the healer functions as a minister of the grace of God by receiving the sick into fellowship and declaring God's mercy to them as much by attitude as by speech or action. Years ago I read a story of a lay person's part in priestly absolution that I have remembered through the years.

A young woman was brought to a hospital after she had been stabbed in a drunken brawl in a disreputable section of the city. All medical care possible was given her, but the case was hopeless. A nurse was asked to sit by the unconscious woman until death came. As the nurse sat looking at the coarse lines on a face so young, the woman opened her eyes and spoke, "I want you to tell me something and tell me straight. Do you think God cares about people like me? Do you think he could forgive anyone as bad as me?" The nurse was hesitant to reply until she had reached out to God for a kind of authorization and reached out toward the injured woman with a feeling of oneness with her. Then, knowing that she spoke in truth, she said, "I am telling you straight. God cares about you, and he forgives you." The woman gave a sigh of relief and slipped back into unconsciousness, and, as she died, the coarse lines disappeared from her face. Something momentous happened between God and that woman through the nurse (21).

The healer-as-minister concept reemphasizes the profound relevance of the message of acceptance. Nonjudging, nondirecting acceptance has a salutary influence on all treatment. This does not mean the suspension of judgment. The ancient biblical principle that the law condemns and destroys if it is not preceded by forgiveness must be at the heart of any healing ministry. The doctrine of justification by grace through faith communicates the good news that one who feels unworthy of being accepted by God can be certain of acceptance.

Meaning Behind Pain and Suffering

Probably the healer as minister has a better chance than many others of understanding the meaning behind pain and suffering.

Pain and suffering may take the form of anxiety and guilt. St. Augustine's view is that anxiety and guilt can be overcome only by God's grace, which is freely given, as stated in his best-known text: *Tu excitas ut laudare te delectet, quia fecisti nos ad te, et inquietum est cor nostrum donec requiescat in te*—"Thou movest man to praise Thee, for Thou hast made us for Thyself and our hearts are restless until they rest in Thee." The message is even clearer in Outler's translation of Augustine's text: "You provide man with the stimulus that makes him want to praise you, because you have made us to be related to you and our inner existence is out of balance until it recovers its balance in right relation with you" (22, p. 93). Similar to Augustine's view is the existential position that there can be no important thinking without self-comprehension. Only by passing through the pain of anxiety and hopelessness can one find a way to faith and truth.

Suffering is a common thread running through the lives of all. Many theologians and philosophers have made it the central problem of their thought and have sought to reorient the individual toward the meaning of life as understood in the meaning of his or her own suffering.

The sensation of pain is generally considered a liability and a burden to physical existence. Although one recognizes the protection pain affords, through functioning as a sentinel or watchman for the living organism, questions arise. Why is pain often disproportionately severe or mild? Why is the type and degree of pain often a hindrance and inhibitor, when reality needs indicate that the danger or peril is not as great as the pain reaction pretends? Pain by most of us is feared next to death, and the awareness of pain begins early in life. Pain is usually considered as synonymous with evil and, if persistent, is compared to a living hell. People usually perceive pain as being a physical phenomenon instead of a mental one, and the psychological component is rarely appreciated.

A major task in the patient with chronic pain is to find some meaning in his or her suffering. One must be clear in one's own feelings about pain before one can help a suffering patient. If one believes there is meaning, despite not being able to find it, one is in a better position to help. Out of long experience with pain, Viktor

Frankl has written: "If there is a meaning in life at all, then there is a meaning in suffering. Suffering is an ineradicable part of life, even as fate and death" (23, p. 67). In Tolstoi's *The Death of Ivan Ilyich*, it was only when Ivan realized the total meaninglessness of his life that he was overwhelmed by the pain of his cancer. As long as there seemed to be a valid meaning to his existence, he could resist the pain and retain both his control and dignity. When he lost the sense of the meaning of his life, he could only scream. Thus, the emotional state determines in large measure the perception of pain and its power over a person.

Kahlil Gibran, in *The Prophet*, has written: "Your pain is the breaking of the shell that encloses your understanding" (24, p. 52). Pain does have the capacity to bring us fully face to face with ourselves and our universe. Dostoevski expressed a basic human concern when he said, "There is only one thing I dread, not to be worthy of my suffering."

The alchemists had a special image for the transformation of suffering and symptom into a value of the soul: the pearl of great price. The pearl begins as a bit of grit, an irritant in one's inside flesh. The grit is coated over day after day until one day it becomes a pearl. Yet it must be fished up from the depths and pried loose. The pearl then is exposed, worn, and open to public view as a virtue. As James Hillman describes the situation: "To get rid of the symptom means to get rid of the chance to gain what may one day be of greatest value, even if at first an unbearable irritant, lowly, and disguised" (25, p. 56).

OUR HERITAGE OF HEALING

Whether thinking in terms of the minister as healer or the healer as minister, one should recognize our heritage of healing as anchored in the biblical tradition. For example, in the New Testament Gospels, one finds as much attention devoted to healing as to any other subject. In studying the biblical healing stories, one discovers certain basic conditions operative in almost all of the cases described. An examination of these conditions will illuminate the guidelines used in a healing ministry and show the similarity between ancient and modern healing and between the approaches of all healers, regardless of vocation.

First, the healing takes place through the activity of an individual or group perceived as having the power and authority to heal. Second, the act of healing often includes the recital of previous healings or other divine events that manifest power for wholeness and transformation. Third, the healing action comes in response to the initiative and request of the sick person, or friends, or relatives. Active desire and expectancy permeate the healing situation. Leslie Weatherhead maintains that a fundamental element in all biblical healing stories is the quality of *expectant trust* (26), and Jerome Frank, in *Persuasion and Healing*, shows expectant trust to be the central thread woven through all healing practices, both ancient and modern (27). Fourth, healing seems to take place in some kind of corporate context, where the group atmosphere becomes a significant factor in the preparation and support of the healing process. Fifth, often the healer employs suggestion and authoritative verbal direction as a part of the healing method. Often the suggestive element is simply the communication of the firm assumption that the ill person will be healed of the illness. Sixth, in many of the biblical stories, physical materials and means are used as an instrumental aspect of the healing action. All six of these basic conditions in healing highlight a heritage worthy of serious study, and remind us that there is more than one factor operative in healing.

CONCLUSION

Some time ago in East Africa, a group of natives, having made a long journey seeking medical care, walked on past a government hospital to reach a mission hospital. When asked why they had walked the extra distance when the government hospital had exactly the same medicine, they replied, "The medicine may be the same but the hands are different" (28, p. 24). In that extra ingredient, symbolized by the hands that are different, may be found an understanding of healing that can color and influence our concept of healing today. In the mission hospital, the minister as healer and the healer as minister lived a common vocation of "each as the other."

Possibly, in the blending of minister as healer and healer as minister, society today could find the kind of "doctor" it really needs for treating its vast array of stress and chronic disorders. Guirdham has suggested that this may be so and that this "new doctor" ought not to resemble the traditional medical doctor but should encompass the concept of the *wise man*. Further, this new doctor or healer must have the knowledge and training of the doctor without medicine's materialism, and the basic attributes of the priest without the paraphernalia. Also, he or she would need the wisdom of the sage (29, p. 150). If we take seriously Guirdham's statement of our need, then we cannot fragment our healing efforts by declaring them spiritual or medical but recognize only the total synchronizing process of healing, for the goal is wholeness and harmony.

Norman Cousins has often spoken of asking Albert Schweitzer what was the essence of the truth he had learned in his lifetime of working with people, as doctor and minister. Schweitzer replied that he had learned that within every person there is a temple and a hospital—the temple for communing directly with all that is high and holy and the hospital to bring healing to the person from within. Schweitzer's work primarily had been to relate to this temple and hospital within his patients.

In recognizing and relating to the temple and the hospital in each human being, the minister and healer declare their kinship in both precept and deed. Nathaniel Hawthorne, although speaking principally of the physician, captures in the following words the true essence of the minister as healer and healer as minister in helping the patient find harmony and wholeness in life:

> If the latter possess native sagacity, and a nameless something more . . . to bring his mind into such affinity with his patient's that this last shall unawares have spoken what he imagines himself only to have thought: If such revelations be acknowledged not so often by an uttered sympathy as by silence, an inarticulate breath, and here and there a word, to indicate that all is understood; if to these qualifications of a confidant be added the advantages afforded by his recognized

character as a physician;—then, at some inevitable moment, will the soul of the sufferer be dissolved and flow forth in a dark but transparent stream, bringing all its mysteries into daylight (30, p. 140).

References

1. Mark 10:45

2. Matthew 20:26–27

3. Tillich P: The meaning of health, in Religion and Medicine. Edited by Belgum D. Ames, Iowa, Iowa State University Press, 1967

4. Nouwen HJ: Creative Ministry. Garden City, New York, Doubleday, 1971

5. Niebuhr HR, Williams DD: The Ministry in Historical Perspective. New York, Harper, 1956

6. Mark 3:15

7. Rimbaud A: A Season in Hell—The Illuminations. Translated by Peschel ER. New York, Oxford University Press, 1973

8. Unamuno M de: Abel Sanchez and Other Stories. Translated by Kerrigan A. Chicago, Regnery, 1956

9. Tosteson DC: Instructions. Presentation of the Tenth Annual Meeting, American Osler Society. Boston, Countway Library of Medicine, April 1980

10. Tillich P: The relation of religion and health, in Healing: Human and Divine. Edited by Doniger S. New York, Association Press, 1957

11. Lain EP: The Therapy of the Word in Classical Antiquity. Edited and translated by Rather LJ, Sharp JM. New Haven, Yale University Press, 1970

12. Plato: Charmides, in The Healing Hand. Edited by Majno G. Cambridge, MA, Harvard University Press, 1975

13. Hamilton E: The Greek Way to Western Civilization. New York, New American Library, 1942

14. Machovec FJ: The cult of Asklipios. Am J Clin Hypn 22:85–90, 1979

15. Williams LP: History and modern medicine, in Implications of History and Ethics to Medicine. Edited by McCullough LB, Morris JP. College Station, Texas, Texas A&M University Press, 1978

16. Engel GL: Too little science: the paradox of modern medicine's crisis. Pharos 39:127–131, 1976

17. Thomas L: The Youngest Science. New York, Viking Press, 1983

18. Benjamin WW: Healing by the fundamentals. N Engl J Med 311:595–597, 1984

19. Maitland DJ: Vocation, in A Handbook of Christian Theology. Cleveland, World Publishing Company, 1958

20. Herrmann N: Go out in Joy. Atlanta, John Knox Press, 1977

21. Horton WM: Our Eternal Contemporary. New York, Harper and Brothers, 1942

22. Outler AC: Anxiety and grace: an Augustinian perspective, in Constructive Aspects of Anxiety. Edited by Hiltner S, Menninger KA. New York, Abingdon Press, 1963

23. Frankl V: From Death Camp to Existentialism. Boston, Beacon Press, 1959

24. Gibran K: The Prophet. New York, Alfred A Knopf, 1923

25. Hillman J: Insearch: Psychology and Religion. New York, Scribners, 1967

26. Weatherhead LD: Psychology, Religion, and Healing. New York, Abingdon Press, 1952

27. Frank J: Persuasion and Healing. New York, Schocken Books, 1974

28. Youngdahl RK: Throughway love. The Lutheran 8:24–25, Dec. 4, 1963

29. Guirdham A: Cosmic Factors in Disease. London, Duckworth and Co, 1963

30. Hawthorne N: The Scarlet Letter. New York, Random House, 1950

5

Religion as Metaphor in Mental Illness

Leon Salzman, M.D.

5

Religion as Metaphor in Mental Illness

Humanity lives in a world of which we are only part master. While knowledge and the advances of science have broadened our command over nature, we are still unable to control completely either ourselves or our environment. We remain dependent on each other's benevolent concern for our survival, and on the impersonal forces of nature, which are entirely outside our control. Uncertainties and insecurities pursue our everyday existence and we have had to settle for some absolutes (such as death) over which we have no control. In more limited ways, we have had to acknowledge our inability to control completely our own functioning—especially in those areas of physiology and psychology that are outside our awareness.

From the earliest records of human behavior it is evident that much activity has been devoted to attempts to control, influence, and guarantee the forces that are beyond man's immediate access. The major content of all primitive religions was devoted to rituals and devices designed to curry favor with the gods in order to prevail upon them for some favorable influence. There were endless ritual practices outside the religious systems, in which the goal was to increase human authority in matters recognized as being not under direct human control. It was simply hoped that a fair exchange could be obtained through such performances. As

humankind's grasp of nature increased, and we developed a grow-
ing confidence in our own strength and power, we developed
more subtle religious practices and more devious devices to guarantee our living. When monotheism replaced polytheism, we did
not apply for as much direct aid but hoped that, because of our
overall devoutness and dedication, God would know and minister
to our needs. Later on, we accepted a ministry, which interposed
with God for us. We made religion less a commercial transaction
and more of a moral commitment. Instead of mere exchange in
the form of sacrifices or gifts, a total devotion in the form of
worship was offered. However, when it came to death, which we
could never deny or overcome, no matter how powerful we became, a different tactic was required. We developed an endless
variety of placating illusions and soporific fantasies of an existence
beyond death that would be even more glorious and fulfilling
than existence on earth. This folklore served many purposes, but
among them was an evasion of the final acknowledgement of
humankind's limited meaningfulness in a physical sense and our
utter incapacity to overcome finiteness. It was an evasion of
powerlessness, and Christian eschatology became a social tranquil-
izer, designed to deal with humanity's inability to accept the
finality of our biological existence. This type of security operation
represented an advance in our intellectual capacities for concep-
tualization.

In view of the role of religion in fulfilling security needs, three
historical periods in the development of religious doctrine and
practices can be distinguished. From the earliest recorded and
extrapolated data, the first phase was mainly pagan, polytheistic,
and largely related to forces of nature beyond one's control and
presumed to be under control of special gods. Worship was largely
ritualistic and opportunistic, and designed to achieve special treatment.

The second phase was a polytheism of gods, who determined all
aspects of one's living, with characteristics resembling humans
with their needs, desires, and petty concerns. Worship was still
opportunistic, but with an infusion of morality and standards,
some of which were humanistic and involved with the average

person, in contrast to the privileged rulers.

The third phase was the development of a monotheistic system, with a godhead who was parental to "all" and concerned with love, regard, warmth, and concern as well as power and authority. This related to the Judeo–Christian tradition, Hinduism, Buddhism, Islam, and similar developments. Worship was directed at achieving goodwill, special treatment after death, and the like.

In my opinion, the role of religion was to enhance one's capacity to deal either with natural or environmental factors beyond one's control or management. Uncertainty, powerlessness, helplessness, and inability to understand any meaning in one's existence demanded both doctrine (with its supporting mythology which varied according to time and place) and ritual (to fulfill the doctrine).

Since the need was omnipresent and insoluble, religious attitudes and orientations were universal, with only rare exceptions as we moved into a time of expanding science, knowledge, and understanding of the world and humankind itself. Only then were there occasioned other modes of achieving security and meaning to present an alternative to religious ideologies.

The advent of psychology, greatly accelerated by Freud, allowed us to examine some of the insecurities and anxieties derived from inner sources rather than from rational or external sources. Freud (1) regarded religion as an "obsessional neurosis," and viewed the rituals as evidence supporting this diagnosis. In my opinion, he put the cart before the horse in failing to note that compulsive behavior, with its rituals, enables a person to have an illusory feeling of control; and therefore, religion (despite its rituals which resemble secular rituals) does not comprise a disease.

A pervasive feeling of helplessness may precipitate large numbers of rituals and phobias as measures of control, including religious metaphors in the form of doctrine and religious practice. Although religion is not a disease, like compulsive defenses it can become pathological when it is excessive, maladaptive, and totally preoccupying. It is a tactic for achieving security and must be viewed as a major device in human functioning with positive, creative, and beneficial consequences. The need and program to fill the need must be viewed from a different perspective when we examine the institution with its political and organizational structure. Of course, they cannot be separated from one another.

Religion is sometimes viewed in psychological circles as an immature, unhealthy, and unrealistic way of confronting the real world with its real problems. While psychotherapists should not attempt to serve as theologians or ministers to their patients, they must be aware of the role of religious feeling in their patients' lives. More specifically, they must be aware of the psychopathological use of religious practices, including scrupulosity and extremism with megalomanias and schizophrenic deteriorations. They must recognize that religious practice may be a metaphor for other problems which directly demand therapeutic involvement. In my opinion, the tendency of psychoanalysts to avoid religious issues relates to their discomfort regarding their own lack of religious feelings, which they (correctly and conscientiously) avoid intruding into the therapy process. On the other hand, religious therapists may be equally uneasy and fail to pursue religious questions for theoretical or technical reasons. Either way it may seem best to stay out of this highly controversial and emotionally charged area. How strange for therapists, who insist that emotional and conflictual issues are their main concern, to avoid such issues!

The study of religions and religious experience has engaged the interest of psychologists as well as theologians for some time. The psychiatrist has had the opportunity to learn a good deal about human behavior in its broader, more spiritual aspects from the theologian, and has been able to give the theologian some significant insights into the motivations of human behavior. The study of religion and religious feelings should include research about dogma, ritual, creeds, history, and liturgy, and also their ethical and human aspects. The phenomena pertaining to religious living and thinking often involve benevolent acts of kindness to one's self and others as well as experiences which fall into questionable areas of psychopathology. Thus, mysticism, fanaticism, stigmatization, flagellation, asceticism, conversion, and religious delusion must be viewed in spiritual terms as well as in psychological terms, in distinguishing between true or constructive religions as opposed to spurious or exploitive religions.

This distinction has been made not so much on the orthodoxy of the beliefs, as on the social and personal consequences of the religion. From this point of view, "spurious religion" could not be characterized as affirming but rather as negating and estranging from reality and one's fellow beings, whereas "true religion" is affirming and is oriented toward objective reality and one's fellow beings in a constructive, benevolent sense.

The problem of religious conversion is of great interest in this regard. The motivation and mechanics of change are involved in the process, which is essentially a phenomenon of change. Religious conversion is a specific instance of the general principle of change in the process of human adaptation. In the process of fulfilling human needs some people follow a rather direct course with minimal strife and turmoil, while others face major obstacles which require major adjustments. These adjustments may constitute constructive, forward-looking change or they may result in regressive movements. Most change—possibly all—is gradual in its development, but since it culminates in a specific moment of alteration or conversion, it may seem to the observer to be an instantaneous, unexplained, mysterious event. However, in every case there has been an incubation or preparation, with lesser or greater struggle, and then a final triggering or precipitating event, or confluence of events, which produces the sudden, dramatic, and obvious change. Where a profound change in philosophy, ideology, or ethics occurs, the hidden but encompassing struggle is especially significant. Thus conversion cannot be regarded as a sudden or dramatic event, although under extremely hazardous and life-endangering circumstances profound changes may occur with only limited background and preparation.

An instance of the significance of religious symbolism and ideology cloaking pathological development occurred in a seminary student, who became violently delusional following some exposure of his homosexual tendencies in a bar near the French Quarter in New Orleans. This episode followed an alcoholic spree after an examination period. He was beaten up by some sailors at the bar. He became delusional and spoke of his stigmata, showing bruises on his hands and forehead. He insisted he was Christ in the Second Coming and documented it by showing his bruises, claiming he was both Jewish and a rabbi. A few days later, after repeated interviews and sedation he was able to identify that he had been beaten up by the sailors because he tried to seduce them. He acknowledged this with horror and shortly thereafter resumed his delusion. He finally came to terms with this experience after several months of treatment.

Paranoid elaborations are very frequent in delusional systems where religious claims or metaphors are used. In these instances the individual feels a particular victim to the outbursts of those who jeer and disclaim the pretension of Christhood. Another example of this occurred in a 35-year-old male, Mr. D. His first paranoid breakdown had occurred at age 26, while he was a theological student. Prior to this he had been an energetic person, full of schemes for the improvement of mankind and preoccupied with his superior, grandiose conception of his abilities and capacities. Periodically he became involved in large-scale adventures based on trivial ideas which he felt would be phenomenal if he could get the proper financial backing. He always expected extravagant returns, with a minimal investment of his time and energy, and based exclusively on his brilliant ideas.

In a manic episode at the seminary, he believed he was Christ and said so, and then proceeded to demand from his colleagues and the administrator the proper recognition for his "Second Coming." The logic for his delusion was interesting. It was based on the fact that he had some Jewish blood and that his mother's name was Maria. In addition, he was born outside of New York, "the capital of the world today," just as Jesus was born near the capital of the early Christian world. He felt his lack of relatedness to his family was also like Jesus. He saw himself as a truly universal man who had a little of everything and was, like Christ, a great lover of humanity. For him, a most significant belief was that Christ, in the Second Coming, would be in the shape of an ordinary man who was little known to the world. In his efforts to secure recognition for his divine self he antagonized the administration, became involved in extravagant dealings, wrote some bad checks, and was eventually hospitalized. During this period of intense activity when he was trying to establish his divinity, he developed many persecutory ideas, particularly that he was being followed. He eventually thought his enemies were trying to kill him. In a later episode he attempted to kill his persecutors, precipitating a second hospitalization. He was released from the hospital when he denied his paranoid ideas and did not mention his belief in his divinity. However, he continued to see himself as Christ for a long time, until the belief was finally questioned and abandoned. What interests us here is the way in which paranoid ideas developed out of his grandiosity. At the onset he thought he felt nothing but love and compassion for his fellow men and the wish to fulfill his mission of universal salvation. Meeting with disbelief, antago-nism, fear, and distrust, he began to assume that there was an organized attempt to deny him his proper role. Well-meaning friends and relatives who attempted to tone down his claims were assumed to be enemy agents, trying to force him to relinquish his divinity. Neighbors and strangers who accidently approached him on the street or in other public places were functioning by design and purpose. Physicians and, finally, the police were enemy agents sent to confuse and destroy him. All this time he was confirming his divinity through a rational and logical examination of his experience. Insignificant conversations with friends and strangers were viewed as tests, which he always successfully overcame. When doubts arose about the reality of his being Christ, he dealt with them easily by insisting that he was not a true son of his parents, but an adopted son, and that the difficulties in being recognized were further proof of his claims. He eventually social-ized his behavior, refrained from mentioning his "true" Christ state, and functioned moderately well until he got involved in more ambitious projects.

This patient demonstrates very clearly the process of formation of delusional ideas. When he was thwarted in fulfilling his grandi-ose claims he presumed an unfriendly reaction designed to deny him his rightful due. It is the sulking, omnipotent demand of the child, who insists on having his wishes fulfilled simply because he demands it, refusing to recognize any realistic limitations. In asking for the moon, he requires that it be delivered to him forthwith and any refusal is equivalent to an unfriendly denial. The paranoid development is an expression of this process in its extreme form, as well as a technique to maintain the underlying grandiosity.

Another illustrative example is E., who came to treatment in a panic state following some fleeting paranoid delusions. Her life was organized around being a dedicated missionary in the field of human relations. After a brief attempt at reorganizing Christian education and attempting to solve the racial problem, she became involved in a dynamically oriented child therapy center, where she was forced to examine the premises of her behavior. This produced panic and a fear of becoming insane, which led her to seek psychoanalytic treatment.

Our relationship developed in an atmosphere in which she would provide me with data about her superior, Christlike devotion to human welfare. She hoped I would reinforce and reaffirm her notions in this regard. While acknowledging that something had gone wrong, she nevertheless expected, through an insight or two over a brief period of time, to overcome these defects so that she could renew her salvation activities. A typical picture unfolded. The patient was notably grandiose. She felt her unique skills and understanding were constantly being hampered by stupid, contemptible people who were selfish and materialistic. She never examined the effect of her behavior on others and she expected them to acknowledge her good will automatically, even while she insulted them. She presumptuously demanded much more from the world than one in her position was entitled to expect. She behaved as though she were the only interested, honest, and unbiased worker, and she could not understand why her activities, which people agreed with in principle, always produced such strong negative reactions. Her suspiciousness was manifest in endless ways, and ultimately was manifested in delusions about being followed, about her telephone being tapped, and about being the object of scrutiny by security agents.

Her father was a prominent figure and public servant in a small western town. He was the leader of all the "good" local causes. His self-righteousness was flavored with truisms and virtuous aphorisms of all kinds; at the same time he was actually recognized for his good works in the community. Everyone, including his wife and children, viewed him as a dedicated, saintly person. E. was convinced early in life that only her commitment to a similar mission in life would satisfy her father. Being the best in her class was fine, but this needed to be accompanied by an unselfish plan to aid humanity as well. Every need, interest, or activity had to be framed in altruistic terms. She was required to be a selfless Christian under all circumstances.

Her activity in therapy paralleled and documented her difficulties in the outside world. She was markedly grandiose, always noble, honest, and dedicated. Her mission was to develop group relationships to ensure peace and good will. She planned to accomplish this through the message she had to deliver, which she expected to be received automatically and accepted. She recognized no exception or difference of opinion, and her behavior had never been examined in terms of its effects on others, as she assumed her views were beyond criticism or objection. Therefore, when there was some disagreement over a program of racial integration, her friends were suddenly perceived as persecutors, who were tapping her telephone, having her followed and investigated, and trying to disgrace her in the community. During the later part of therapy, she said: "Most of my insecurities were handled by considering myself a great leader, a 'superman' type of character. My behavior went along with this. I established a position as leader of a peer group and worked hard to maintain this position, often putting family responsibilities in the background in order to do this. I used the role of martyr to act out deep feelings of being unfairly treated and rejected. . . . The idea of competition . . . the idea I am living with and working with people more mature and wiser than I am, is impossible to digest even though I can cheerfully recognize such a situation." In pursuing her grandiose claims she idealized the "superman" and derogated all evidence of weakness and inadequacy in herself and others.

Love and dependent relationships were dangerous and detestable to her, since they implied weakness. In a letter to me, she wrote: "It isn't my fault. It is that Goddamned Salzman's fault . . . He is helping me to learn to be dependent. He is forcing me. He has broken my spirit. He has tamed me. He is going to force me to complete helplessness. That is why I am so tense. I have lost and I can't acknowledge this reality. I have lost. But I can't lose. I have never lost. It is impossible. I won't believe it."

The maintenance of this grandiose immunity from being human was necessary to prevent what the patient felt would be the extreme opposite, that of utter helplessness and contemptuous failure. The patient was compelled to demand automatic acceptance and avoid a realistic appraisal of her activities. Otherwise, she would have needed to face the picture of her imperfect humanness and destroy the grandiose defense system. All her standards, ideals, and activities were of the extreme Utopian order, which could not be compromised in the slightest. In therapy, every awareness was met by an immediate need to resolve the difficulty instantly and for all time. The obvious incapacity to do so produced outbreaks of anxiety, panic, and paranoid accusations.

The paranoid development follows a program which cannot be fulfilled unless the person is actually hailed as a savior, and which consequently meets rebuff and rejection by the environment. Suspicion, hostility, contempt, lack of trust, and delusional formulations are an attempt to guard and guarantee the grandiosity. Such patients expect automatic acceptance. They trust only in magic and they quickly learn to distrust the world, which is engaged in a massive scheme to seduce, weaken, and destroy them.

The therapeutic skills which are needed to deal with any paranoid development require a thorough understanding of the adaptational value of such a defense. The paranoid process is designed to support an integration based on the notion of one's grandiose uniqueness, total independence, and omnipotent and omniscient capacities. It stems from a deep sense of personal inadequacy and a danger of meaninglessness in accepting any insignificant evidence of personal deficiency. Tenderness, closeness, intimacy, and dependency are totally unacceptable, since these qualities indicate weakness and less than superhuman potentiality. The need for absolute power and magical performance, divorced from realistic effort, necessitates total control over the environment. Manipulation and exploration are accidental accompaniments and are needed to guarantee the fulfillment of the patient's mission. Playing God, or being God, often means being king and peasant both at the same time. The discrepancies and contradictions in these extremes are rarely noted. The grandiosity gets expressed in terms of a mission or a supreme dedication to fulfill the Savior role— whether as a dedicated humanist, an invincible prophet, or a brilliant scientist, scholar, or diplomat.

It is apparent that not all paranoid persons have messianic missionary goals or humanitarian concerns. However, behind every grandiose claim which characterizes this personality disorder—whether it be an insistent demand that one is always right (omniscient), or that one gets exactly what one wants (omnipotent), or simply that one has superior esthetic, artistic, or scientific talents—lies the feeling that one has a special mission and personal uniqueness and significance.

Such noble and easily justifiable projects make the defense almost invincible. How can such an ideal or goal be minimized? Obviously, it is not the goal which is questioned, but the basis for its existence, and the means used to achieve it. The attempts to fulfill the grandiosity are all compulsive and involve an enormous amount of anxiety which appears in every aspect of living. This all-pervasive anxiety is at the core of the difficulty and central in the therapeutic handling of this process.

The externalization or projections are the secondary effects of the person's attempt to carry the grandiose tasks into fulfillment. The environment, in not recognizing the supreme genius of the individual, tends to minimize, disparage, or overlook it, which is the greatest misfortune that can befall a paranoid. To deal with these possible consequences in a real world, an elaborate system of persecutory delusions, or ideas of reference, develops.

Treatment of the paranoid will often demonstrate neurotic difficulties involving religious manifestations. In every instance it is an error for the psychotherapist to get involved in theological discussions of dogma or ritual. Such questions belong in the realm of the theologian. However, it may often be necessary to allow the patient to relate his or her religious background and beliefs as they manifest themselves in the mental disorder. The therapist's role is to investigate how the therapist is used in the defensive elaborations of characterological distortions, rather than to take some moral stance on the validity of the theological concepts.

The resolution of the paranoid distortions can only occur when they are dealt with in a direct confrontation of reality in an atmosphere already partially open to confrontation. The following vignette demonstrates this process. I first saw A. during a quiet period in his illness when he was unable to go to work. He was being supported by his wife because no job worthy of his status was being offered him. Besides, at any time the call might come, acknowledging his "Second Coming," and he was holding himself ready for it. During the seven months I had been seeing him, he attempted to examine his living with respect to the major facets of his personality: his grandiosity, his contempt for the deficiencies and weaknesses of others, and, particularly, his special significance as a multigenius who would be acknowledged and given his true reward.

At one interview, he described a piece of rumination about a device he had worked out to get larger rockets off the ground, which would beat the Russians and save the government millions of dollars. He would be awarded the medal of honor and the Nobel prize, as well as a fabulous reward. This device would use steam as a propellant, as is done on aircraft carriers to propel planes off the deck. I responded to this by saying very emphatically that his presumption had assumed fantastic proportions. I said that he was presuming to solve a problem that was currently being tackled by the most eminent scientists in the world, experts in rocketry who had probably devised steam propulsion for airplanes, and who are now spending all their time and energy and skill in trying to solve this problem. Yet, through a brilliant insight of 10 minutes spent in casual consideration, he—who knew nothing whatever about this subject—had devised a solution. I elaborated and emphasized the immensity of his lack of humility. A. attempted to defend his position by giving examples of other brilliant discoveries that had occurred in just this way and finally said he did not mean it seriously, anyway.

At the next hour, he arrived in excellent spirits and described the hour-long ride home after his last session, and the intervening four days. He said that at first he had been furious. Then he resolved to prove his point by developing the mechanism. Finally, he had to agree that I had been right. He recognized that all his life had been a succession of just such grandiose schemes, some of which he had tried to actualize, with disastrous consequences. He added that no one had ever confronted him with the enormity of his distortions in this way before; others had tried to tone him down, argue with his scheme, or say nothing and just humor him. It was a real comeuppance, which he recognized had been coming to him for some time. He said he now understood why he thought he was Christ; he assumed he was omniscient and omnipotent and only Christ combined such virtues. He finally felt that he no longer needed to be Christ and instead could go ahead with a project he had organized recently with some friends. He was convinced that he had broken the hold which the delusions had on him; he no longer felt that television cameras were following him all the time, and he thought that perhaps he did not really need to be a big shot.

Certainly the issue is not finally resolved when an awareness, even as striking as this, occurs. It is really only the beginning of therapy, for now the way is open to investigate what necessitated the development of such a grandiose device to avoid humiliation and failure. Harry Stack Sullivan (2) believed that when patients work through one parataxic distortion there is the possibility of favorable outcome.

SCRUPULOSITY

The extremes of guaranteed controls in a religious sense are manifested in the disorder of scrupulosity. In this compulsively driven behavior, the individual hopes to achieve a guaranteed, certain accounting with God by performing the ritual with an unquestioned devoutness (for example, 10 Hail Marys becomes 100, and every ritual is repeated 10- or more-fold to accentuate the sincerity). This is clearly a disorder, and is acknowledged as such by established religion as well as by psychiatrists. Such extreme behavior to achieve a guaranteed outcome can be an embarrassment to religious groups as well as a destructive, disorganizing activity for the individual. This phenomenon is a compulsive symptom in an obsessive–compulsive neurosis. Such persons may be so precise in their pursuit of the ritual or so perfectionistic in their religious life that they become "holier than the Pope," and are critical of the priesthood and its practices. The use of religion as a metaphor for the expression of compulsive requirements is determined by the developmental relationship to religious experiences in one's maturation. In addition, the availability of absolutes in a godhead allows the ritual to have an added quality of control. Consequently, the treatment of scrupulosity is identical to that of the therapy of other obsessive–compulsive states (3). Here, too, the theology is secondary, while the issue of control must be the primary object of therapeutic concern.

Scrupulosity is a direct manifestation of the influence of religion in a psychiatric disorder. Yet its significance is not religious but psychopathological—a defense mechanism against powerlessness and helplessness in the human condition.

References

1. Freud S: Obsessive Actions and Religious Practices (1907), in Complete Psychological Works, Standard Edition, vol. 9. Translated and edited by Strachey J. London, Hogarth Press, 1959

2. Sullivan HS: Obsessionalism, in Clinical Studies in Psychiatry. New York, WW Norton, 1956

3. Salzman L: Treatment of the Obsessional Personality. New York, Jason Aronson, 1980

6

How to Evaluate Patients' Religious Ideation

Ruth Tiffany Barnhouse, M.D., Th.M.

6

How to Evaluate Patients' Religious Ideation

Religious language is sometimes extremely difficult to evaluate. Nor is this difficult for psychiatrists only. Clergy are also likely to err. In general, psychiatrists tend to be too suspicious of it, many believing that all religious language is tinged with pathology. Clergy may make the obverse error of taking it at face value, failing to note when the religious terminology is cloaking an underlying mental disorder. This paper will first consider the nature and function of religious language and then describe some ways of discriminating between appropriate and pathological uses of it.

THE NATURE AND FUNCTION OF RELIGIOUS LANGUAGE

Much contemporary language theory dismisses religious language as meaningless on the grounds that it is not falsifiable. But this rests on the assumption that only scientific statements have meaning, using Karl Popper's criterion of falsifiability to distinguish science from nonscience. Paul Ricoeur, a philosopher who has written extensively about both psychoanalysis and religion, disputes this view. He defends "natural language," citing the German linguist Von Humboldt's definition of language as "an infinite use of finite means." Religious language, says Ricoeur, belongs to the sphere of natural language, and its strength lies in the fact that all its terms are polysemic—for every sign there is more than one meaning. "The strength of a polysemic language resides in its sensibility to contexts" (1, p. 94).

The language used in psychotherapy is also polysemic. Any analytically oriented therapist knows that the language patients use means far more than they realize consciously, and much of the therapeutic task is to get patients to recognize the multivalence of what they have said. This is because the presenting symptoms stand for those aspects of the patient's meanings which have been repressed. At the same time, the patient's language may also contain the creative possibilities for improvement. As Ricoeur says, "indeterminacy and creative power appear to be wholly inseparable" (1, p. 94). This means that when patients have been helped to recognize the indeterminacy and multivalence of their own statements, not only can they deal with their pathological meanings by admitting them to consciousness rather than by symptom formation, but their own creative and healing potential can be unleashed and new directions chosen for their life.

Religious language, which is intrinsically symbolic and metaphorical, operates on precisely the same principle. Ricoeur says that "metaphor is one of the strategies thanks to which language is compelled to transgress its previous limits, and becomes able to bring to language the not yet said" (1, p. 94). If only because it deals with the unknown, religion is much concerned with the "not yet said." This has to do with the underlying function of religion, which is to provide what may be called *cosmic orientation*.

As psychiatrists, we are accustomed to evaluating people's mental stability in terms of the accuracy of their orientation to time, place, and person. In a precisely similar way, religious health depends on the answer to the same questions posed on a cosmic scale. How does one perceive oneself in relation to time with a capital T, all the time there is—Eternity? What is one's place in the total scheme of the universe? Who is one, in relation to all of this? There is no known culture, however primitive, which has not evolved at least rudimentary answers to those questions. And

there is no person, however isolated or individualistic, who has
not considered them. The set of answers which anyone has arrived at, with or without reflection, and in however limited or
negative a way, constitutes that person's religion. As William
James remarked about a young atheist at Harvard, "He believes in
No-God and worships Him." One is dealing here with that which
is in principle unknowable, at least in terms of any modern
definitions of knowledge. The fact that *all* human beings consider
these questions is therefore all the more remarkable.

Some philosophical and psychological theories make claims
about such questions, if only to declare that the traditional transcendent formulations of the religions are mere epiphenomena of
the human psyche. Such declarations are not denials of religion,
they *are* a religion, since they make a claim about the ultimate
system of orientation (2).

According to this general definition, theology is a subset of
religion. Each of the many theologies is a symbol system, usually
highly elaborate, through which its adherents attempt to deal
with the mystery of the Unknowable, and to tolerate its para-
doxes. Theology has two components: the symbols themselves,
and the speculations, whether official or private, about their im-
port. Christianity and some of the other "high religions" have
more than one official system of interpretation of the basic set of
symbols. In terms of this symbolism, believers answer the questions of meaning and purpose, sometimes using their own interpretations but often relying on the pronouncements of religious
authorities. (The term *high religions* refers to those which have a
large number of adherents, and which have endured for centuries.
These are Buddhism, Christianity, Confucianism, Hinduism, Islam, Judaism, and Taoism) (3).

Attention has often been drawn to the common use of religion
through the ages, in giving believers a sense of control of their
circumstances and destiny, whether that control be real or illusory. Many rituals, both in primitive and in high religions, have
been interpreted as magical rites designed to propitiate the god(s),
either to secure personal advantage or to avert disaster. There is no
doubt that religion has often been used that way, and still is by

many people. It is, however, a primitive use and does not encompass what religion means to persons of any degree of spiritual maturity. The underlying function of providing cosmic orientation is far more important, even in primitive religions, than gaining a feeling of control, important as that may be to some individuals. One example is the practice in Native American religions of arranging the "sacred space" in which rituals are performed as a model of the universe. This depends on the concept that the microcosm of the human scale reflects, at least ideally, the macrocosm of the universe. It is believed that, by intentionally performing ceremonies in such sacred space, a connection can be made with cosmic forces. The architecture of Gothic churches whose floor plan is in the shape of a cross reflects a similar idea.

Rather than using religion to gain a feeling of control, mature believers have the opposite idea, that of relinquishing egoistically based control (4). Through the practice of religion they try to discern what their proper place is in the overall Cosmic Design, believing that their particular gifts and talents are to be used in the service of facilitating some inscrutable future harmony which transcends the finiteness of human limitations. It is obvious that a strong ethical sense of obligation to one's fellows will develop when such beliefs are firmly held. The ethical behavior of less-mature believers will be based on the instructions of religious authorities. Naturally these authorities are subject to the whole range of human fallibility, including the contamination of madness. Examples of the effect of that fallibility might include Pope John Paul's stance on birth control but would certainly include the tragedy of Jim Jones and the Guyana massacre.

The suspicion, ripening to certainty, that one is not, and cannot be, in control of the cosmos—nearly always accompanied by the equally strong suspicion that Something or Someone is somehow in charge—is evidently constitutive of human consciousness, since some expression of that idea has characterized every known society. In fact, the claim that one does have such control is always and everywhere understood to be delusional. The idea that there may be Nothing or No-one in charge, that the cosmos is just somehow there, is extremely new. It is so new that it is only during this century that any society has adopted it as an official plank of its organizational platform with any degree of success. But even those who hold such views believe in something beyond themselves, such as the laws of nature or the findings of science, to which questions about the unknown must be referred and whose known principles cannot be flouted with impunity.

It is too early to tell whether these new developments represent hubris or enlightenment. It may even be that they are merely a variant of religious language, a variant so new and apparently strange that its continuity with the known religious vocabularies has yet to be recognized. It would not be the first time in history that those who discovered a new symbol system believed that it was a literal description of reality.

Such efforts toward cosmic orientation exclusively through conscious rationality must, however, explain the ubiquity of religion. Freud's view that the concepts of God and the Devil are "nothing but" the projection of good and bad paternal imagoes is a well-known instance. Rizzuto's recent research has confirmed the occurrence of such projections while demonstrating that they include imagoes not only of the father but always also of the mother (5). Subtle students of religion agree that such projections take place. However, far from seeing them as a "nothing but" explanation of God, they see them as a serious hindrance to the real purposes of the spiritual life. Ulanov succinctly describes the process of peeling away these anthropomorphic hindrances in her article, "What Do We Think People Are Doing When They Pray?" (6).

Even in the most advanced rational systems, further unknowns, perhaps even unknowables, are continually being discovered. Nevertheless, the modern mind faithfully believes that all can eventually be comprehended, or else tries to assume that what lies beyond the grasp of the human sensory–intellectual apparatus can for practical purposes be safely ignored. The advantages of the Enlightenment to civilization in general and consciousness in particular cannot be denied, but it is dangerous to be stuck in it. Both the dangers and the advantages have been elegantly discussed by Owen Barfield in his erudite book on the nature of thought and experience in relation to the evolution of consciousness (7).

The exclusively rational mindset as an ideal is grounded in the comfortable precisions of a Newtonian universe. But the physics of the last 70 years has shown these precisions to be primitive illusions. The new knowledge has not yet begun to inform our daily lives or to affect the way medicine is taught and practiced (8). Yet the quantum universe we actually live in is one where nothing is real, where we know nothing about what is happening unless we are actually watching, where ordinary ideas of causality have no meaning, where there are 10 (or possibly 11) dimensions, where there are many worlds—perhaps an infinite number— which exist "sideways across time from our reality, parallel to our own universe" (9, p. 235). As if that weren't enough, for all our sophisticated understanding of biology we know nothing, absolutely nothing, about volition, whether conscious or unconscious, not even about the simple act of will required to raise a finger (10).

The existence of realities beyond those immediately obvious is one of the oldest religious intuitions. We can now see the application to conventionally religious language of Ricoeur's previously quoted statement that "metaphor is one of the strategies thanks to which language is compelled to transgress its previous limits, and becomes able to bring to language the not yet said." It has always been necessary to have some way of referring to that which lies beyond the realms which can be rationally understood or manipulated. Such ways have varied, and still do, over a wide range of styles. Some are extremely primitive, some concrete, some superstitious, some admitting the nonrational only in a logical emergency, some abstract, some extremely sophisticated. All are characterized by the presence of metaphor and symbolism, whether the believer recognizes that fact or not.

For example, many conservative Protestant fundamentalists, who take the Bible literally, vigorously deny that there is anything metaphorical or symbolic about their religious beliefs. This is at least partly because they have grown up in an age which values scientific rationality and "hard facts" above other forms and ways of knowledge. They are applying to the field of religion the same mindset that has allowed some linguistic philosophers to assert seriously that propositions which are unfalsifiable are meaningless. Other philosophers have concluded that such claims are empirically absurd, and refute them in elegant and dignified language. Ordinary people are more likely to adduce the fact that such statements as "I love you" are not meaningless, even though they are not subject to proof. But when it comes to the beliefs and images which importantly govern their lives, many contemporary people cannot tolerate any suggestion that these might not be incontrovertibly true. Therefore they are driven to concretize their religious symbols in order to be able to think of them as "real facts."

They do not realize that this maneuver spells death to any truly religious outlook or expression. As the Episcopal theologian Urban Holmes has said, "[Biblical] literalism is a modern heresy—perhaps the only heresy invented in modern times" (11, p. 13). This is because such extreme concretization tends to prevent the exercise of one of religion's important functions, which is to keep believers in right relation to the Unknown and the Unknowable. When religion is doing its proper job, it helps people to steer a constructive middle course between two destructive extremes.

One extreme can be expressed in a statement such as this: "I know exactly what God has in mind for the whole universe. To be sure, God knows more than I do, but he has told me his plans for me and for all humanity. I therefore have the right to condemn all who do not agree with me." Religious fanatics fall into this camp, along with all ideological extremists, many of whom are atheists. The other extreme goes something like this: "Everything is meaningless, or at least incomprehensible. I am so insignificant in the total scheme of things that it can't matter what I do." This attitude is unlikely in serious adherents of any of the Western religions but is quite common in those who have lost their faith or who never had any. Such an attitude can lead to apathy and despair, or in other cases to narcissistic libertinism. From the psychiatric point of view, either extreme is pathological and can manifest in either neurotic or psychotic forms. From the religious point of view, either extreme is perverse, if only because it prevents sufferers from the exercise of responsibility to others or from the development of their own best possibilities. (There are, of course, people who manage to avoid these extremes without the support of a theological system.)

From the standpoint of society, either of these extremes held by a sufficiently large number of people carries serious dangers. Jung pointed out that people need to have a reference point outside the self and transcending the human plane, in order to avoid being at the mercy of the collective lowest common denominator, and/or the State or other tyrannical authority. He says: "It is possible to have an attitude to the external conditions of life only when there is a point of reference outside them. The religions give, or claim to give, such a standpoint, thereby enabling the individual to exercise his judgment and power of decision" (12, p. 19). If one actually has such an attitude, one has the courage to be in the minority—even at great personal peril, if need be. One also has the humility to realize that being in the majority is no guarantee of being right. It is undoubtedly true that many practitioners of religion, ordained as well as lay, fall short of this ideal, which is a difficult one to live up to consistently. But all of the high religions give, along with the symbolic language, specific instructions on what the practical fruits of true belief will be, and these always include respectful regard for self and others.

As we have seen, ego-inflation can take two forms, fancying oneself to be superior to all others or utterly insignificant. But if in order to avoid such inflation it is necessary to have a balanced cosmic orientation, how is this to be accomplished? Few if any are able to do so in purely abstract terms. The natural way seems to be to do it through images. The psychiatric practice of dream inter-pretation depends heavily on the natural tendency of the human psyche to express in image and symbol not only those things which it chooses to forget, but also those future creative possibil-ities which are still embryonic. As therapists, seeing those who have not managed their lives adequately, we may sometimes forget how important dreams are in those whose mental health is robust. It has been demonstrated that pathology develops very quickly in people who are prevented from dreaming. Dream im-ages, whether consciously attended to or not, apparently serve to balance and fill out those conscious attitudes which are too one-sided for optimal function. Both normal and psychotic persons often use dream symbols identical to those in religions they know nothing about, and symbols and mythological cosmic speculations are often remarkably similar from one religious system to another. It appears that the sacred mythologies of the various religions are to the human race as dreams are to individuals. We should seriously consider the possibility that mythological deprivation may have effects just as unfortunate for society as dream deprivation does for individuals. This may shed some light on the fact that, historically, the decline of religion has been accompanied by serious social disorder.

HOW TO DISTINGUISH APPROPRIATE FROM PATHOLOGICAL USES OF RELIGION

Immature uses of religion do not necessarily imply psychopathology even when, from the religious point of view, they may properly be considered evidence of spiritual pathology. To put this idea another way, the psychiatric frame of reference is more limited than that of religion. For example, all instances of selfishness are evidence of disordered religion but they are not all evidence of psychopathology, even though some may be, such as narcissistic character disorder. Nevertheless, in the presence of certain kinds of religious immaturity it can be very difficult to determine whether or not the religious language used by the patient is in fact psychopathological.

Therapists attempting to evaluate patients' use of religion need to consider the following questions. What is the patient's stage of faith development? What is the religious history? What is the patient's social response to the religious experience? Is religion being misused as a resistance to therapy?

Building on the work of Piaget, Erikson, and Kohlberg, Fowler has shown that religious development takes place in stages, and that these appear in an invariant order (13). Stage 2 is characteristic of school children though it is sometimes seen in adolescents and adults. In this stage everything is taken literally and symbols are

one-dimensional. Some primitive forms of fundamentalism encourage believers to get stuck at this stage. It is rare for these people
to seek psychotherapy since their religion usually forbids it. They
may see all mental and emotional disorder as diabolically originated and therefore subject only to religious healing. But occasionally they do end up in therapy and their use of religious language
can make it very difficult to determine whether or not they are
psychotic. An interview with such a person in treatment for
obsessive–compulsive disorder might go something like this:

Patient: "I can't help myself. The devil puts doubts in my mind and
            I have to go back in the house six times to make sure I've
            turned off the gas."
Doctor: "Always six times?"
Patient: "I pray. Sometimes God answers my prayer and speaks to
            me. He tells me to wash my hands to cleanse myself from
            sin. So I do. I always do that seven times. Seven is the perfect
            number, you know, so that's what God tells me to do.
            Sometimes he lets me off with only three washings, one
            each for Father, Son, and Holy Ghost. Those times God's
            voice is sweet and forgiving, but when I have to wash seven
            times his voice is angry."

In subsequent discussion the patient is unable to describe the
problem in other terms or to accept alternative formulations of the
meaning of the experience.

If the anamnesis has included a religious history, some light
may be shed on the problem. Patients should always be asked in
what religion, if any, they were brought up. Answers such as
Protestant, Catholic, or Jewish are not sufficient. Which Protestant
denomination? If Catholic, did they attend parochial schools?
What kind of religious training was given by the nuns or priests? If
Jewish, was the family Orthodox, Conservative, or Reformed?
Were the parents assiduous in religious practice or not? If only one
parent was religious, how was that handled in the family? Does
the patient practice any religion now? If they have changed from
the religion of childhood, abandoned religion altogether, or taken
it up for the first time, what were the circumstances of the
change? How often do they attend services? Do they find religion
supportive? Do they find it frightening? What effect do their

beliefs have on the way they conduct their daily life? Have they consulted their pastor or rabbi about their problem? If so, what did he or she say? What is their idea of God, whether they accept or reject that idea? The research instruments of Rizzuto and Fowler can be helpful in eliciting the answers to many of these questions, particularly the last one (5, 13).

Knowing these answers makes the evaluation of conversations such as the one reported above much easier. If the patient is a lifelong member of a primitive fundamentalist sect, *in the absence of other signs* it is safe to assume, at least provisionally, that he or she is not psychotic. Should a patient who is Roman Catholic or a member of one of the mainline denominations such as Presbyterian, Methodist, Lutheran, or Episcopalian report symptoms the same way, the index of suspicion of psychosis would be much higher. This is partly because these churches do not support fixation at Fowler's Stage 2. Should a Unitarian or a Quaker talk like that, the diagnosis of psychosis could be automatic since members of these groups tend to be at least at Stage 4, and since such language isn't even an arcane part of their symbolism.

The presentation of such an extreme case was deliberate, to make the point that the pathological significance of religious language can seldom be determined by immediate context alone. One must always ascertain the cultural and religious context of the statements, and a familiarity with Fowler's faith-stage theory will also be extremely helpful. Although cases of Stage 2 are rare, persons in Stages 3, 4, and 5 will frequently be seen in therapy.

Stage 3 is typical of adolescents, but many adults have stopped here. It is a conformist stage, highly dependent on the opinions and judgments of significant others. Such people have an ideology, but since they have not objectified it for examination they are unaware of it as such. "Authority is located in the incumbents of traditional authority role . . . or in the consensus of a valued group" (13, p. 173). Most, but not all, conservative fundamentalists are in this stage. But there are many adherents of mainline Protestant denominations as well as many Roman Catholics in this stage also.

Stage 4 develops appropriately in young adults, but many do not reach it until their 30s or 40s. This is a demythologizing stage, in which the capacity for critical reflection on one's identity and ideology is developed. Rationality, however defined and however well or poorly practiced, is highly prized. A great many people remain at this stage within their religious institutions. But it is also characteristic of the educated secular classes who have abandoned traditional theological symbols but retain speculation about meaning and ethics and a strong sense of social responsibility. A serious problem is that people at this stage tend to feel superior not only to people in earlier stages but also to those who have gone on to Stage 5. The prevailing cultural value placed on science as the royal road to all knowledge is characteristic here. The large majority of psychiatrists are in this stage, which contributes to the common problems of understanding many kinds of religious language.

When the transition to Stage 5 occurs, it is precipitated by " . . . disillusionment with one's compromises and recognition that life is more complex than Stage 4's logic of clear distinctions and abstract concepts can comprehend" (p. 187). It is conjunctive, using a both/and way of thinking rather than either/or. It is characterized by what Ricoeur calls "second naivete" in which symbolic power is reunited with conceptual meaning (1). It is at home with paradox, with truth in contradictions, able to reconcile the opposites in mind and experience. It is open to the strange truths of others. Reaching this stage is rare before midlife. We need not concern ourselves with Stage 6, since it is extremely rare, achieved only by a saintly few.

Such statements as "God spoke to me . . . " or "I saw the Virgin Mary . . . " may, of course, indicate hallucination or delusion at any stage. It is important not to jump to this conclusion, but to get a detailed description of the experience. It may become obvious at once whether, however vivid, the patient knows the experience is not real in the ordinary sense of that term. Stage 4 people generally clarify that at once. But, for Stage 3 people, the customary religious metaphors may be so ingrained that the distinction may be harder to make. The biggest trap for the diagnostician can be the failure to distinguish between Stage 2 or 3 and Stage 5, since persons at all of those stages may be either unwilling or unable to express their religious views except in the symbolic terms of their faith. Stage 2 people cling to such language because for them such language *is* reality. Stage 3 people may cling to such language because to abandon it feels like abandoning the truth of their religion. For them, such language is the only way they know to talk about spiritual reality. Stage 5 people are more likely to feel that to express themselves in everyday language does violence to the numinous quality of their experience which can only be approximated through religious symbols. For them, such language is the best way of describing *one* kind of reality. The possibility of confusion is well exemplified by a Stage 4 psychiatrist I know who, after reading Jung's autobiography, concluded that he must have been an ambulatory schizophrenic all his life! In making the distinction, evaluation of how the patient functions in modes other than the religious is helpful, since people are usually consistent. It is also helpful to know whether the patient has participated in any of the secular or religious systems now providing training in *guided imagery* since that will affect the way they experience and describe psychological states. Questioning should clarify the difference between such effects, ordinary consciousness, and pathology.

The next step is to find out *in detail* what the patient thinks an appropriate response to the voice or vision might be. Psychotic responses are highly idiosyncratic, usually having to do with the self, others being involved only in a paranoid way. Normal responses are in the direction of healthier self-understanding, better relations with others, or constructive action of some sort.

But not all abuses of religious language are psychotic. Neurotic uses must also be identified. Is the sense of guilt out of proportion? Patients may use a punitive interpretation of religion as resistance to avoid dealing with the underlying issue. Some patients may say "I have committed the sin against the Holy Ghost." This is from a mysterious passage which simply says that the sin against the Holy Ghost is the only one that cannot be forgiven, but what that sin is is not specified. It therefore makes a very handy hook for the projection of guilt. Occasionally patients will misuse the religious concept of forgiveness to deny feelings of guilt.

Do the religious concerns cause consistent subjective discomfort? If so, the likelihood of a neurotic contaminant is higher, even if the content of the religious concern sounds appropriate. Many people use religion as resistance to therapy. It is important to recognize that it is not their religion which makes them do this. I know of cases where psychiatrists, recognizing such a problem, have tried to handle it by weaning the patient away from religion. This is unwise. There should be no hesitation to label such a misuse of religion—even in some cases to suggest that they consult their pastor or rabbi. In fact, such abuse of religion is a common reason for clergy to refer parishioners to psychiatrists. Dealing with the underlying problem will improve not only the patient's mental health, but will contribute to spiritual maturity as well.

It should be recognized that an unsolved religious problem may contribute to emotional ill-health. I learned this early in my residency when a hospitalized psychotic woman insisted for months that there was something she could tell no psychiatrist but needed to confess to a priest. In desperation, I finally called one, who was the Professor of Pastoral Care at a local seminary. He heard her formal confession, told me only that she did indeed have something substantive to confess. The patient improved at once and within two weeks was ready for discharge. This is a dramatic example, but similar things can occur with non-psychotic outpatients.

Psychiatrists who know very little about religion would do well to study it (3, 14). Sex and religion are, in some form, universal components of human experience. No psychiatrist would dream of trying to practice without knowing a great deal about sex. It must be recognized that religious concerns, in whatever language they may be expressed, cannot be irrelevant to therapy if they are brought up by the patient. The task is to understand whether they are being used as a smokescreen for something else, or whether they are an important component of the patient's healthy functioning.

References

1. Ricoeur P: The Biblical worldview and philosophy. National Institute for Campus Ministry Journal for Jews and Christians in Higher Education 6:91–111, 1981

2. Barnhouse RT: Spiritual direction and psychotherapy. The Journal of Pastoral Care 33:149–163, 1979

3. Smith H: The Religions of Man. New York, Harper & Row, 1958

4. Jung CG: Transformation Symbolism in the Mass, in Psychology and Religion: West and East. Princeton, Princeton University Press, 1969

5. Rizzuto A: The Birth of the Living God. Chicago, University of Chicago Press, 1979

6. Ulanov AB: What do we think people are doing when they pray? Anglican Theological Review 60:387–398, 1978

7. Barfield O: Saving the Appearances. New York, Harcourt, Brace, and World, 1965

8. Dossey L: Space, Time, and Medicine. Boulder, Colorado, Shambhala Publications, 1982

9. Gribbin J: In Search of Schrödinger's Cat: Quantum Physics and Reality. New York, Bantam Books, 1984

10. Green EE, Green AM: Biofeedback and states of consciousness, in Handbook of Altered States of Consciousness. Edited by Wolman B, Ullman M. New York, Van Nostrand Reinhold (in press)

11. Holmes UT: A History of Christian Spirituality. New York, Seabury Press, 1980

12. Jung CG: The Undiscovered Self. Boston, Little, Brown, and Co., 1958

13. Fowler JW: Stages of Faith. San Francisco, Harper & Row, 1981

14. Ulanov A, Ulanov B: Religion and the Unconscious. Philadelphia, Westminster Press, 1975

7

Religious Concepts in Psychotherapies

Sidney Werkman, M.D.

7

Religious Concepts in Psychotherapies

This appears to be a time of profound soul-searching in psycho-analysis—a situation not unknown to religions both in the past and the present. The preceding chapters of this monograph confirm the importance of reviewing the state of psychoanalysis and its relationship to religion, and carry the process of examination forward with insight, respect, and charm.

Dr. Robinson, in Chapters 1 and 2, highlights the need for new ideas, new collaborations, a disenthralling of ourselves from previous views in this transitional period when psychoanalysis has lost the outstanding intellectual position it enjoyed after the Second World War. Dr. Knight, in Chapters 3 and 4, emphasizes the importance of an awareness of our own imperfections and problems and, in fact, the possibility that we might delight in them and gain from them, as we work with patients. He poignantly brings our attention to the problem of the priest without faith who, nevertheless, continues to minister to his believing congregation. We might extrapolate from this example the issue of the therapist whose earlier confidence in a particular psychotherapeutic school has had to be modified. Dr. Salzman, in Chapter 5, describes techniques of working with exaggerations and distortions of religious thoughts and concepts in disturbed religionists. Dr. Barnhouse, in Chapter 6, delineates the language of both fields, describing how pathology arises from developmental issues and distortions. Her guide to how to take a religious history is a model to be followed.

The contributions to this monograph probe the psychoanalytic ideas that began in the glow of a powerful 19th-century medical research focus on the experimental and scientific methods. Much of the writing in psychoanalysis (and other psychotherapies, as they relate to psychoanalysis) assumes that psychoanalysis is a field of science. But that assumption is now in the process of a re-examination that recognizes the religious and philosophic ideas from which analysis arose and with which it is still entwined. Dr. Robinson, in an excellent earlier paper,"The Illusion of No Future: Psychoanalysis and Religion," described that theme clearly. She quoted Apolito, who wrote "Freud tore down one religion to build another one, in some ways even more fanciful and mysterious than the one of which he disapproved" (1, p. 213). And Dr. Robinson then added her own wise appraisal of religion: "Countless generations have found in religion a source of inspiration and comfort—a Weltanschauung which contributes to an orientation in time and space and some understanding of what it means to be a conscious creature in the universe" (p. 222).

A deep, poignant theme of disenchantment and a striving for redefinition runs through the preceding chapters and emphasizes the value of comparing some fundamental concepts contained in both religion and psychoanalysis. As they have been uneasy partners on numerous occasions, from the time of *Malleus Maleficarum* and witch burnings, it may be of interest to note similarities and differences in the two fields that illuminate aspects of each. I will not attempt to make judgments about the power or efficacy of either one, but rather to sketch something of the qualities they share and the differences they reflect (see Table 1).

Historically, religion has been the path taken by those seeking significant answers to inner problems. Though religions have been by no means silent on social and political issues, they characteristically evolve from a concern with the relationship of mankind and God. Religion takes all of life as its province. The adap-

Table 1. Fundamental Concepts in Religion and Psychoanalysis

Psychoanalysis	Religion	
The individual	Relationship to society and to God	
Relief of *DSM-III* symptoms	Forgiveness	Reconciliation
Ordinary human misery	Systems of Faith and Belief	

tive viability of religion is indisputable.

Psychotherapy has become, for certain groups in contemporary Western society, the court of first resort for the resolution of personal and interpersonal psychological concerns, taking over much of the territory assigned to religion in the past. Though the two-person engagement is but a small part of the purview of religion, psychotherapy is carried out primarily in this arena. It is directed toward the alleviation of inner, subjective distress through a confidential relationship between therapist and patient that utilizes speech, thought, reason, feeling, and fantasy to explore and modify inner experience and to restructure disturbed outward behavior. The sometimes tautological diagnostic labels in the field—emotional disorder, inner conflicts, marital problems, anxiety reactions, psychiatric illness—reflect a state of some confusion and disorder as well as hoped-for creative solutions. The rich profusion of definitions and goals to be found in both religions and psychotherapies run parallel to each other. Both fields are in a constant process of redefinition, refinement, and transformation (2).

Psychotherapeutic treatment is concerned with the individual and a "self." Its aim is to help the patient "feel better," to be more comfortable, and to experience wellness and wholeness. Though the results of psychotherapy might well include a decrease in symptoms and "better" relationships with spouse, children, and others, the major goal is a subjective inner experience of goodness or health and a decrease of inner conflict. That catchphrase goal of psychoanalysis, to change neurotic symptoms into ordinary (that is, conscious) human misery, does not offer any prescription about how the patient is to live after treatment. Just as a surgeon cannot authoritatively prescribe for the human condition after a successful appendectomy, so the analyst and the body of psychoanalytic thought offer no encompassing plans for a good life. Thus, psychotherapy is directed toward the understanding and improvement of inner states and personal functioning. Its effect on others is a secondary result.

Religion takes as its field, not only the self, but in a far more important sense, the individual's relationship to society and to God. These concerns take precedence over personal gains that might accrue from individual feelings of pleasure, comfort, or satisfaction. Religionists frequently choose paths of pain, humiliation, suffering, and even martyrdom and death in the service of their religion. They often turn from the pursuit of sexual pleasure, personal gain, individual satisfaction, or comfort in order to live up to fundamental religious beliefs that are thought to be inherent in human beings. When psychotherapies make profound statements about human experience without experimental confirmation they tread on the ground of religion.

Many of the ideas used in psychotherapy have evolved from those of religion, some overtly and other implicitly. In some ways psychotherapy might be seen as a subset, a special case of religious ideation. Some examples follow. Obviously they could be expanded greatly—and argued passionately—but it is important to recognize the kinship of psychotherapy and religion (see Table 2).

SOME ELEMENTS SHARED BY RELIGIONS AND PSYCHOTHERAPIES

Sacred Scripture

For thousands of years the Old and New Testaments of the Bible, the sayings of the Buddha, the Koran, and the Hindu Vedas have spoken authoritatively to the problems of humankind. Most issues of life, relationships, conflicts, death, meaning, and hope have been considered and refined in such scriptures, though the conclusions and prescriptions vary from one belief system to another. These writings form a powerful encyclopedia of anthropology and treatment. In a similar way, the Standard Edition of the

Table 2. Religious Elements in Psychotherapies

Sacred scripture and esoteric knowledge
Relationship to founder
Priest(ess)hood
Focus on life-transition issues and rites
Concern with cosmos: systems of belief and faith

---

works of Freud have taken on, for some, a dimension of sacredness. These writings have been annotated with commentaries and used as solemn, authoritative references in discussions of psychotherapy. The writings of certain other psychoanalysts have gained a similar stature, and can be compared to Paul's Letters in the the New Testament, in the way that both make the transition from a person to a movement.

Esoteric Knowledge and Mystery

A threat of meditation, contemplation, trance, altered states of consciousness, and transfiguration runs through religion and promises secret knowledge to the initiated or elected. Though altered states of consciousness, the use of hypnosis, and the concept of transference are integral to the psychotherapeutic encounter, they do not rise to the same level of highly organized mystery material known to religion. However both seem to promise, explicitly or inferentially, secret knowledge available only to the elected.

Relationship to Founder

Founders, whether religious or psychological, tend to be deified by followers, whether they wish such elevation or not. Religions are strewn with examples of founders who asked that a cult of personality or deity not be developed around them. Yet this very deification occurred. The same tendency can be seen in the psychoanalytic movement, in the iconic photographs of Freud that have been displayed in the stylized psychoanalytic offices of the last 40 years.

Priest(ess)hood

The progression of study and acceptance into an inner circle with a set-apart status, characteristic of priesthoods, is paralleled in psychoanalysis by the various levels of candidacy and acceptance into a training institute and professional association. A psychoanalytic institute candidate shares many of the exaltations and trials of the novice in a religious order.

Life-Transition Issues

Religions have evolved organized rituals for dealing with life-transition issues—career choice, marriage, the understanding and resolving of conflicts, the resolution of guilt, the anxiety of illness, and the reality of death. Each of these issues has become integrated into one or another form of psychotherapy, and life-stage theorists and therapists abound (3, 4).

Cosmos

Religions tell humanity of an orderly, harmonious, systematic universe, one that is meaningful rather than chaotic. They offer total answers, a "cosmic orientation," for human situations and promise ultimate meaning even when the individual is unable to recognize that meaning. Systems of faith and belief aim to strengthen this sense of cosmic meaningfulness. Psychotherapies tend to flirt with similar concepts, especially when the power and significance of the therapies are most strongly challenged.

It is in the definition and resolution of sin and non-neurotic guilt that religions have their greatest strength, and psychotherapies appear to be weakest. The psychotherapist who entreats one to forgive one's self can offer few techniques to effect that self-forgiveness. Religions have evolved well-defined ways to resolve sin and guilt through the expression of sorrow in a community context followed by ritualized restitution and forgiveness. Whenever a psychotherapist takes on such a burden in the treatment situation, it is a curious question as to how guilt is resolved. Is it possible that the therapist does, however unwittingly, play God?

Even from these glimpses of issues shared by religions and psychotherapies, it should be clear that similar issues and concepts energize both. In many of the issues described it would be fruitless to try to describe where one field ends and the other begins. Fortunately, a recent group of research findings in neurobiology and psychopharmacology have begun to function as powerful probes to clarify the language of both religion and psychotherapy. Some of these findings and the concepts they illuminate follow.

Both psychotherapy and religion assume that the individual can use a *mind*, often conceptualized as the cerebral cortex, to think and reason. Yet many types of disturbed functioning (schizophrenia, depression) are being recognized as syndromes that develop from deep-brain structures, essentially divorced from thinking and consciousness, structures that can be little affected by psychological motivation. It may be that we are, indeed, more determined by physical and physiological properties than psychological systems have wished us to believe in the past.

We have little control over certain aspects of "affect" and "feeling" that derive from primitive midbrain and limbic system structures that have changed little over millions of years of evolution. Complex, altricial bonding, nurturing behavior, and even "love" derive, in part, from hypothalamic and limbic system phenomena that first arose in lower mammals.

The experiences of awe and mystical union have a long history in religions. Euphoria and states of ecstasy, even transfiguration, occupy significant niches in religious scripture and ritual. Some complements of the mystical state include the following: a sense of revealed meaning to the initiated person, meaning that may be indescribable in words but nevertheless deeply experienced. In the mystical state there may be a sense of union with infinite power, a passive giving up of the will and abandonment of the self. A feeling of timelessness and perfection may ensue. Following the mystical experience—and this is what separates it from psychopathological states—there is a return to the ordinary world as a changed, transformed person with a new sense of authority and direction that is utilized in societal action. A harmonious new integration that solves personal problems in a permanent fashion is experienced.

Though many of the terms differ, psychotherapies frequently define their goals in similar terms. The resolution of personal problems, a sense of empowerment, a harmonious new integration, and experience of transformation and integration are typical terms that express psychotherapeutic effectiveness (5).

We now know that experiences of awe, mystical union, and ecstasy can be triggered with some reliability by newly discovered neurotransmittors—endorphins, catecholamines, and neuropeptides—that produce and modulate states of joy and hope that had previously been the province of religion and, more recently, of certain psychotherapies. It may be that the potential for experiencing such states is an innate human characteristic, just as the ability to smell with exquisite precision is a built-in capability of rodents and other lower animals.

Humanity's Faustian romance with the meaning of life, the attempt to find direction and a personally guiding principle in the universe, may reside not only in a religious spirit, but in the constantly evolving development of the human brain. Though psychotherapies typically eschew any pretence to giving meaning to life, a deeper study of their underlying principles will often demonstrate that they implicitly do just that. This is not to criticize them, but to recognize that the search for meaning seems to be inherent in the human brain. As Suzanne Langer (6) reminded us, just as the bird is an organism that flies, Man is a symbol-transforming organism. Our brains are made to construct meaning, to develop reasonable conceptualizations, whether they are scientifically correct or not (7). Thus, many of the conceptualizations that were satisfying until the recent revolution of research in neurobiology no longer carry powerful explanatory value. Many other examples could be brought to bear to show that neuroscience and neurobiological experiment have chipped away at concepts cherished most by religions and psychologies.

One area that contemporary neuroscience has sidestepped is that of subjective consciousness. All those qualities of inner awareness and inner state that are seemingly impervious to experimental scientific study form the main strength of religions and even of psychotherapies. It may be that subjective consciousness will persist as the perennial domain of religion and, perhaps, psychotherapy. Subjective consciousness is also the pathway to art and music and to all the cultural phenomena that appear to make life worthwhile after the brain and the body make it possible.

Obviously, as in all important discussions, no one answer will suffice. This is a time for questioning, for seeking new directions. What the authors of this monograph suggest is that the traffic that has flowed from religion to psychoanalysis and psychotherapy might well turn backward, toward an attempt to understand the structure of religious interfaces with psychotherapies, as well as forward into the realm of neurosciences. This may be a time when psychotherapy can be enriched by a sophisticated study of anthropology and religion through the development of courses on the structure of belief systems given by sophisticated, committed religionists.

The two fields need to know when they borrow from each other, indeed, when they become each other, and how they can help each other. And both can profit from recognizing the inroads being made in their domains by neurobiological research.

References

1. Robinson LH: The illusion of no future: psychoanalysis and religion. J Am Acad Psychoanal 13:211–228, 1985

2. Meissner WW: Psychoanalysis and Religious Experience. New Haven, Yale University Press, 1984

3. Erikson EH: Identity, Youth, and Crisis. New York, WW Norton, 1968

4. Levinson DJ: The Seasons of a Man's Life. New York, Knopf, 1978

5. Wallace ER: Freud's mysticism and its psychodynamic determinants. Bull Menninger Clin 42:203–222, 1978

6. Langer S: Philosophy in a New Key. Cambridge, Harvard University Press, 1957

7. Turner VW: The Forest of Symbols. Ithaca, Cornell University Press, 1967

8

Dialogue of the Future

Klaus D. Hoppe, M.D., Ph.D.

8

Dialogue of the Future

In the framework of this monograph and on the basis of the contributions of Drs. Robinson, Knight, Salzman, and Barnhouse, there is the rare opportunity of presenting the relationship between psychiatry and religion as a dialogue of the future. Such dialogue occurs not only between theology and psychiatry, philosophy and psychoanalysis, but also arises from a new understanding of brain functions and neuropsychology. Thus, modern men and women, hovering on the "dividing line between bliss and logos" (1), may regain faith in themselves as images of God.

HEMISPHERIC SPECIALIZATION

In the 1960s and early 1970s, a small number of humans who suffered from intractable epileptic seizures had complete cerebral commissurotomies (that is, the two cerebral hemispheres were surgically disconnected by sectioning the corpus callosum and the anterior commissure). Apart from being helped by this operation, these commissurotomy, or split-brain, people provided an opportunity to examine the two cerebral hemispheres separately and to clarify their functions.

Using special testing procedures (2), it could be confirmed that (in right-handed people) the left hemisphere is specialized for comprehension and production of speech, as well as for a mode of information processing that is linear, analytic, systematic, sequential, objective, nonrepresentational, and externally focused.

The right hemisphere is not devoid of speech, as it plays a role in speech intonation, gesture, and expressive speech. On its part, the right hemisphere is specialized for the melodic and chord progression of music, the perception and manipulation of spatial relations of and between objects, and for visual constructive tasks. More generally, the right hemisphere is specialized for a mode of information processing that is nonlinear, synthetic, structural, simultaneous, subjective, representational, and internally focused. The right hemisphere senses the forest, so to speak, while the left hemisphere often cannot see it for the trees.

A scientific meeting, The Dual Brain: Hemispheric Specialization in the Human, at UCLA in January 1984 revealed that the original concept proved valid, especially also in nonoperated people.

CLINICAL OBSERVATIONS

Twelve Commissurotomy (Split-Brain) Patients

Stimulated by the original findings of Sperry and Bogen (3), I interviewed 12 commissurotomy patients and their relatives. Apart from life history, mental status, psychodynamics, and psychosocial situation, I focused upon dreams, fantasies, and their ability to form symbols. The examination of five female and seven male split-brain individuals, all but one of them right-handed, and between the ages of 21 and 50 years old, revealed a paucity of dreams, fantasies, and symbols. The dreams lacked condensation, displacement, and symbolization; the fantasies were unimaginative, tied to reality, and utilitarian; the symbolization was concretistic, discursive, and rigid (4). These clinical observations were confirmed by psychological tests (5) and an independent scoring by Hoppe and Bogen (6).

Experimental Study

In order to evaluate these clinical observations, an experimental study was performed by TenHouten and colleagues (7–11). Eight cerebral commissurotomy patients were paired with eight normal control subjects. The pairs of subjects were matched for age, sex, right-handedness, ethnicity, language spoken, and order of language learning, as well as community of residence.

The stimulus for the experiment was a film, *Memories: If Truncated in Mourning*, which intends to symbolize death and loss. The meaning of the film is conveyed only by music and by visual images; the major events are shown not directly but symbolically.

In the first scene, a baby plays in its crib. Then the crib is shown without the baby, and the death of the baby is symbolized by a slowing of the piano music ("Somewhere over the Rainbow"), and by a white bird slowing in its rotation over the empty crib. The second scene has a similar theme. A boy is swinging in a park, he kicks his ball away, and chases it into the street. A car approaches, the ball is seen rolling into the street, and then the street and swing are empty. The death of the boy is symbolized by the slowing of the piano music ("Raindrops Keep Falling on My Head") and by the slowing, empty swing, while the camera zooms towards the shadow under the swing. There are no spoken words in the film.

If the significant meaning of the symbols is grasped by the subjects, then the film is apt to invoke feelings of sadness, loss, separation, and death. The film was shown individually to each of the 16 subjects four times, and a total of 20 questions was asked after each showing.

We found that commissurotomy patients tended not to use affect-laden words, whereas they applied auxiliary verbs to excess, which is associated with the passive and indirect presentation of themselves. They tended to use incomplete sentences, being especially prone to leave out the subject or other important part, and applied adjectives sparsely, exhibiting a speech that was dull, uninvolved, flat, and lacking color. A test of group differences in factor score showed the commissurotomy subjects to be alexithymic;

that is, they lack the ability to verbalize feelings and fantasies (12, 13).

With regard to the six Sifneos questions used clinically before (6), commissurotomy patients significantly tended to deny fantasies and symbols, and either did not recognize or did not interpret these symbols. In addition, they were prone to describe the circumstances surrounding events, but not their own feelings about these events.

A qualitative global analysis showed that the split-brain patients symbolized in a discursive, logically articulated structure, using mainly a secondary process (as opposed to a presentational structure) as an expression of a predominantly primary process. They also showed a concreteness of symbolization, emphasized dense rather than creative capacity, lacked a summary of the whole gestalt, showed a relatively impoverished fantasy life, and tended not to be able to convey symbolic meanings.

The following diagram may illuminate the different forms of symbolization in the two hemispheres when stimulated by a film full of symbols and feelings. According to Susan Langer (14), discursive symbolization is articulated and needs a secondary thought process, the reality principle of Sigmund Freud (15). Presentational symbolization represents the logic of feelings as expressed in fine art, mystical experiences, or music, and exhibits primary-process attributes, such as condensation and displacement.

According to Luria (16), the right frontal lobe is involved in the perceptual analysis of semantic images of a series of pictures that depict the stages of a story, and in the cognitive representation of the expressive elements of these images. The right temporal area is known to be involved in the grasp of the significance of visual images and music.

In expressive people, the presentational symbolization and imagery in the right hemisphere is transferred to the left hemisphere via the corpus callosum. I call this transformational process of verbalizing presentational symbols *symbollexia*. In the left hemisphere, symbols and images are comprehended and verbalized in the Wernicke and Broca areas. Between these two speech centers,

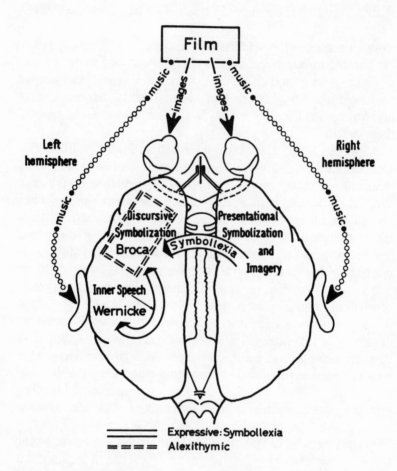

Figure 1. Symbollexia. Discursive and presentational symbolization.

neuronal connections and centers for speech encoding facilitate a process of inner speech. As we could see, commissurotomy patients lack symbollexia. Their predominantly discursive symbolization in the left hemisphere corresponds with alexithymia in people who are nonoperated but function in a similar way. I call it *functional commissurotomy*, or *isolated cerebral lateralization*, and found it in survivors of severe persecution (17) and also in

some Catholic priests (18). Alexithymia is also described in patients with psychosomatic and somatoform disorders, psychogenic
pain, and substance-use disorders (19). A recent article in *OMNI*
(20) estimated that 10 percent of the population in the United
States may be alexithymic.

Feelings

Thus, alexithymia can be understood as disrupted communication between the hemispheres due to the inhibition of symbollexia and inner speech, as well as a lack of verbalized feelings. The
source of our affects and emotions is located in deeper brain areas,
the limbic system. Especially in the hypothalamus are found
"rewarding" regions with emotional or affective reactions, as well
as pain-related regions (21).

Bryden and Ley (22) have found that emotional stimuli are
perceived more accurately when presented to the right hemisphere, which suggests that the right hemisphere has a special and
prominent influence on the reception and expression of emotions.

Presentational symbolization and imagery is closely linked with
feelings. In contrast, exclusive discursive symbolization is prone to
become arid, concrete, and rigid. Symbols are changed into signs
which have lost their emotional meaning, and which replace
warm communication, vitality, and spontaneity. In contrast to
symbols, signs are one-to-one relations in which denotations prevail over connotations. Especially obsessive–compulsive people
separate themselves from emotional experiences by objectifying
their world experiences via signs. Very often, this impoverishment of symbolization and feelings leads to an impoverishment of
interpersonal relationships and disrupted communication with
the world around one's self (23, 24).

Resymbolization and Second Naiveté

On the basis of these neuro-physiological and -psychological
findings and concepts, it is understandable that resymbolization is

not only a psychotherapeutic goal (18). The whole area of spirituality is involved. The German theologians and psychoanalysts Scharfenberg and Kaempfer (25) symbolized Biblical stories and founded a symbolic-communication group for clergy. In this country, Louis Savary in his cassettes, "Praying from the Right Brain," pointed to the rich symbolic imagery of Jesus' parables and in Ignatius of Loyola's spiritual exercises.

If we replace the stimulus film in the diagram with the experience of liturgy, the spiritual meaning of symbollexia and inner speech (praying) becomes evident. If the cross is not experienced as a tree of life planted on Calvary, or as the throne of love, then God may be really dead for too many people in our Western world, who are only operating and communicating with signs. Resymbolization means the retrieval of meaning through the development of what Paul Ricoeur (26) has called "second" or "post-critical naiveté"; that is, openness to wonder and faith.

The contribution of this field of neuroscience is to show how a first naiveté of original presentational symbols, imagery, and feelings may be transformed via symbollexia to verbalization or inner speech and into a second naiveté which is beyond the exclusive use of discursive symbolization. The new knowledge of functions and presentations in our brain can be understood as a dialectic process: from the thesis of original feelings, images, and presentational symbols in the right brain, via symbollexia through the antithesis of left-brain activities, to the synthesis of a second naiveté which faithfully accepts spiritual and religious experiences.

Such an understanding of a bridge between brain and mind, mind and spirituality, corresponds with Robinson's complementary approach to psychoanalysis and religion, and with Barnhouse's symbolic–metaphorical language of religion, which brings to language "the not yet said." It corresponds with Salzman's chapter on religion as metaphor of mental illnesses and, I might add: not only illnesses, but all mental processes. My concept of symbollexia is illuminated by Knight's chapter which contains marvelous metaphors and imagery; for example, an operation as an enactment of the Biblical story of Jonah and the whale.

The Matrix of Ability to Believe

If we conceptualize, with Ana Maria Rizzuto (27), object representations as "representing, remembering, fantasizing, interpreting, and integrating experiences with others," we understand not only the rich complexity of them and the dialectic connection with self-representations and the immortality of these memories,

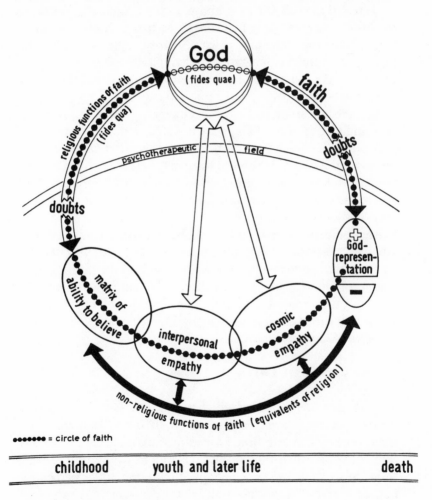

Figure 2. God–representation.

but we can also appreciate the crucial role of presentational symbolization, imagery, and symbollexia.

The matrix of the ability to believe is very early given in human life. Winnicott (28) pointed out that the eyes and the entire face of the mother are the child's first mirror. Later on, this experience becomes the first representation of God, whose mirroring function is reflected in the biblical account of creation: "So God created man in His own image, in the image of God created He him" (Genesis 1:27). Eye contact as first indication of symbolization creates transitional space. If basic trust (29), sufficient parental mirroring, or separation–individuation (30) of the original grandiose–narcissistic self (31) are lacking, the matrix of the ability to believe is deranged.

The precursors of superego development: imitation, idealization, and identification (32)—may be molded into an "inner master" (punitive conscience and benevolent ego-ideal) who enslaves the self and is equated with the voice of God (18). In the process of individual development, interpersonal and cosmic empathy may restore the God-representation and basic trust and thus counteract religious doubts.

As the diagram shows, matrix of ability to believe and interpersonal and cosmic empathy might be effective in atheists who are using nonreligious functions of faith—for example, in their veneration of Lenin in his tomb at the Red Square in Moscow. As much as they may idolize him as a God-like figure, however, Lenin will never become God because he lacks the transcendent qualities of God.

The Circle of Faith

Kierkegaard (33) understood that to know God, to approach him, requires a "leap," a suspension of one's inevitable self-centeredness. The leap from brain functions and mind to God is more profound than the "mysterious leap from the mind to the body" (p. 4), since by our functions of faith (*fides qua*) we believe in the content of faith (*fides quae*), defined as metaphysical entity and ontological–ethical priority (34). The functions of faith com-

bine intellect with emotions, thinking with feelings; that is, left-
and right-hemispheric thinking, especially symbollexia.

As I have learned from 50 psychodynamically oriented psychotherapies with Catholic clergy over the last 12 years, a fruitful
area of cooperation between psychotherapists and priests becomes
evident in the intertwined relationship of immanent God-representation with the transcendent idea of God. Doubts in God-
representations, caused by derangements of matrix or empathy,
can be treated in the psychotherapeutic field, whereas doubts of
faith in God need the help of a spiritual director. Constant feed-
backs between interpersonal–cosmic empathy and God sustain
and strengthen the circle of faith.

It seems to me that the concept of God-representation, and circle
of faith, has been illuminated by the foregoing chapters. Salzman
spoke of the developmental relationship to religious experiences in
one's maturation. Barnhouse focused on cosmic orientation and
the danger of mythological deprivation. Robinson described similarities and differences between spiritual directors and psychoanalysts. And Knight spoke of the wound of empathy with the
patient, and pointed out that doctors and spiritual directors may
become pilgrims with others on the path to healing. These authors seem to have taken to heart the wisdom of Albert Einstein:
"I assert that the cosmic religious experience is the strongest and
noblest driving force behind scientific research" (35, p. 425). They
have engaged in a dialogue of the future which includes knowledge and understanding of brain functions and neuropsychology,
and affirms that the view "psychiatry and religion have no future" is an illusion (36).

References

1. Ricoeur P: Hermeneutik und Psychoanalyse. München, Kösel, 1974

2. Sperry R, Gazzaniga M, Bogen J: Interhemispheric relationship: the
   neocortical commissures: syndromes of hemispheric disconnection,
   in Handbook of Clinical Neurology. Amsterdam, North–Holland,
   1969

3. Bogen J: The callosal syndromes, in Clinical Neuropsychology. Edited by Heilman K, Valenstein E. New York, Oxford University Press, 1985

4. Hoppe K: Split-brains and psychoanalysis. Psychoanal Q 46:220–244, 1977

5. Hoppe K: Split-brain: psychoanalytic findings and hypotheses. J Am Acad Psychoanal 6:193–213, 1978

6. Hoppe K, Bogen J: Alexithymia in twelve commissurotomized patients. Psychother Psychosom 28:148–155, 1977

7. TenHouten W, Hoppe K, Bogen J, et al: Alexithymia: an experimental study of cerebral comissurotomy patients and normal controls. Am J Psychiatry (in press)

8. TenHouten W, Hoppe K, Bogen J, et al: Alexithymia and the split brain, I: lexical content analysis. Psychother Psychosom 43:202–208, 1985

9. TenHouten W, Hoppe K, Bogen J, et al: Alexithymia and the split brain, II: sentential content analysis. Psychother Psychosom 44:1–5, 1986

10. TenHouten W, Hoppe K, Bogen J, et al: Alexithymia and the split brain, III: global content analysis of fantasy and symbolization. Psychother Psychosom (in press)

11. TenHouten W, Hoppe K, Bogen J, et al: Psychosomatic personality structure in the split brain: Gottschalk–Gleser content analysis. Psychother Psychosom (in press)

12. Sifneos P: The prevalence of "alexithymic" characteristics in psychosomatic patients. Psychother Psychosom 22:255–263, 1973

13. Nemiah J: Alexithymia. Psychother Psychosom 28:199–206, 1977

14. Langer S: Philosophy in a New Key. Cambridge, Harvard University Press, 1942

15. Freud S: Formulations on the two principles of mental functioning, in Complete Psychological Works, Standard Edition, vol. 12. Translated and edited by Strachey J. London, Hogarth Press, 1958

16. Luria A: Higher Cortical Functions in Man. New York, Basic Books, 1967

17. Hoppe K: Severed ties, in Psychoanalytic Reflections on the Holocaust: Selected Essays. Edited by Luel SA, Marcus P. New York, KTAV Publishing House, 1984

18. Hoppe K: Psychoanalysis and Christian religion: past views and new findings. Bulletin of the National Guild of Catholic Psychiatrists 30:30–42, 1984

19. Taylor G: Alexithymia: concept, measurement and implications for treatment. Am J Psychiatry 141:720–732, 1984

20. Huyghe P: Speechless mind. OMNI, March 1984:26, 96

21. Isaacson R: The Limbic System. New York, Plenum, 1982

22. Bryden MP, Ley RG: Right-hemispheric involvement in the perception and expression of emotions in normal humans, in Neuropsychology of Human Emotions. Edited by Heilman KM, Satz P. New York, Guilford Press, 1983

23. Lorenzer A: Die Wahrheit der Psychoanalytischen Erkenntnis. Frankfurt, Suhrkamp, 1974

24. Hoppe K: Destruction–reconstruction of language and forms of interaction: clinical aspects of Lorenzer's concepts. Contemporary Psychoanalysis 13:52–63, 1977

25. Scharfenberg J, Kaempfer H: Mit Symbolen Leben, Olten, Walter, 1980

26. Olson A: Myths, Symbol, and Reality. London, University of Notre Dame Press, 1980

27. Rizzuto AM: The Birth of the Living God. Chicago, University of Chicago Press, 1979

28. Winnicott D: Playing and Reality. New York, Basic Books, 1971

29. Erikson E: Childhood and Society. New York, WW Norton, 1963

30. Mahler M, Pine F, Bergman A: The Psychological Birth of the Human Infant. New York, Basic Books, 1975

31. Kohut H: The Analysis of the Self. New York, International Universities Press, 1975

32. Spitz R: On the genesis of superego components. Psychoanal Study Child 13:375–404, 1958

33. Coles R: Erik Erikson: The Growth of His Work. Boston, Little Brown and Co., 1970

34. Deutsch F: On the Mysterious Leap from the Mind to the Body. New York, International Universities Press, 1959

35. Clark RW: Einstein: The Life and Times. New York, The World Publishing Co., 1971

36. Robinson LH: The illusion of no future: psychoanalysis and religion. J Am Acad Psychoanal 13:311–328, 1985

9

Religious Contexts for Change in Sexual Orientation

E. Mansell Pattison, M.D.
Gala S. Durrance, M.Ed.

9

Religious Contexts for Change in Sexual Orientation

Religion and sexuality have a long history of interrelatedness. Sexual metaphor, symbolism, rite, and ritual are frequent components of many religious systems. On the other hand, religion as a construction of social reality and behavior has typically framed a culture's definition of the meaning of sexuality and the appropriate parameters of sexual behavior.

In recent years there has been considerable religious debate on the topic of homosexuality, as framed within Western Judeo–Christian religious traditions. Some religious groups have advocated the adoption of homosexual practices and life styles as religiously desirable alternatives, including the development of homosexual churches. Other groups have attacked homosexual practices and life styles as antireligious, and eschewed any attempt to link religious life to homosexual persons. Thus, there has been political, social, and ideological polarization around homosexuality as a religious issue.

Part of this debate revolves around the empirical question of whether a homosexual orientation is an unchangeable attribute or is subject to change to heterosexual orientation. Often this empirical question has been debated as an ideological/political issue, as if debate would solve the empirical scientific issue. And indeed, there are substantial social implications embedded in the empirical problem. If a homosexual orientation is immutable and fixed, what does that imply for the societal valuation of homosexuality? Conversely, if homosexual orientation is variable, mutable, and alterable, a different set of social implications obtain.

For many years, the standard psychiatric view was that homosexual orientation represented a maldevelopment in psychosocial identity, and consequently a variety of interventions were employed to change sexual orientation, ranging from hormonal treatment, to behavioral modification, to psychoanalysis. This view has more recently been challenged on several counts. First, homosexual orientation has been redefined by some as a normal variant of human sexuality. Second, the idea of intervention or treatment of homosexual orientation as a pathology has been disavowed. Third, the goals of psychological intervention in some treatment programs have been to make homosexual orientation, behavior, and life style positive desiderata.

The above polar antitheses among clinicians in the mental health fields again fail to address the empirical question of mutability of sexual orientation. Thus, the mental health debate parallels the religious debate, and both intertwine with each other.

A felicitous experiment of nature presented itself several years ago with the emergence of a self-help movement, termed the ex-Gay movement. This is of some interest because it is a religiously based movement that partakes of both the religious and mental health fields. In brief, members of this movement seek to offer religiously oriented ministries to homosexual persons. The movement accepts a homosexual orientation as a human situation that does not preclude religious affiliation, commitment, and participation. Yet, at the same time, the movement does not support homosexual behavior and homosexual lifestyles. Members of the ex-Gay movement have claimed that participants in their religiously oriented self-help programs have changed sexual orientation. If empirically established, those findings would have potential significance for our understanding of the phenomenon of sexual orientation, per se, as well as direct implications for the mental health field in terms of the goals of interventions with homosexual persons.

In this Chapter, we present survey data on the claimed change in sexual orientation among members of the ex-Gay movement. The substantive findings are modest and inconclusive. The more important issue is that the data raise further substantive questions about how sexual orientation develops, is maintained, and may change. These latter questions will be reviewed in our final discussion, in relation to current anthropological research.

ISSUES OF SEXUAL ORIENTATION

The *development*, *maintenance*, and *change* of sexual orientation are issues of substantial theoretical and clinical interest. Sexual-object choice appears to be a very complex social behavior which encompasses a gamut of heterosexual and homosexual phenomena.

A Kinsey Institute report (1) on the *development* or "path" to adult homosexual behavior demonstrates that homosexual preference and behavior is strongly linked to the formation of gender identity; that homosexual orientation is psychologically established in childhood; and that adult homosexual behavior is the continuation and culmination of that childhood psychosexual propensity.

Their data suggest that an exclusively homosexual orientation is tightly linked to identity and thus highly impervious to change in response to adolescent and adult social learning. In turn, an exclusively heterosexual orientation is probably just as impervious to change. A bisexual orientation appears more amenable to change in either a heterosexual or homosexual direction.

A critical review by Gadpaille (2) offers further clues. First, interference with early childhood sexual expression and experience increases the likelihood of preferential homosexuality and of sexual dysfunctions and disorders generally. Second, there is evolutionary and neurophysiological evidence for an innate heterosexual bias. Preferential homosexuality is not found naturally in any infrahuman mammalian species. Third, homosexual activity per se, even in the extreme case of cultures that institutionalize a period of exclusive homosexuality in adolescence, will not compromise the ultimate change to exclusive heterosexuality if there are clear cultural definitions and expectations of *gender-dimorphic roles*, which reinforce the innate heterosexual bias.

This latter process is documented by Herdt (3) in a New Guinea highland tribe with ritualized universal male homosexuality. At about age eight, all boys are taken from the home and strictly segregated from the young girls. They live in a central hut and serve as passive homosexual partners to older youths. At about age 15, the males then become the active, dominant homosexual partners to younger boys. The homosexual practice is religiously ritualized and practiced in secret. At about age 20, each male then marries a preselected woman. A traditional, monogamous, heterosexual family is established. Only rarely is this pattern broken, and a male who retains homosexual identity and practice is severely condemned, and ostracized from the tribe. In this study we see the powerful effects of dimorphic socialization, even though the process includes a period of universal male homosexual behavior in the culture.

Problems of *maintenance* of sexual orientation are documented in the situational or contextual homosexual behavior seen in prisons or in the military (4). Culturally institutionalized gender roles and sexual behavior are also seen in temple prostitutes and palace eunuchs, or in a culturally required homosexual role for actors, shamans, warriors, etc. (5). It would appear that individual sexual preference can be overridden by social availability, social role, or social demand for a specific gender-role identity and/or sexual behavior.

Third is the issue of *change* in sexual orientation. Persons of *bisexual* orientation do fluctuate in the direction and intensity of their sexual orientation. Their preference of psychosexual choice and sexual behavior appears relatively malleable to social contextual constraints and opportunities. However, Altshuler (6) has recently argued that sexual orientation is *dichotomous* rather than a *continuum*. He does not view bisexuality as a midpoint, but rather as a way station toward either a homosexual or heterosexual orientation.

More problematic is the issue of change in those of lifelong exclusive sexual orientation. Based on Gadpaille's observations, we might expect the exclusively heterosexual to be impervious to change. Yet we know that heterosexuals in social isolation, as in prison, may behave as exclusive homosexuals for many years. Further, a common clinical phenomenon is change to homosexual orientation during regressive phases of intensive psychotherapy. Thus sexual orientation may not be nearly such a "fixed" state as we commonly assume. Change from exclusively homosexual to exclusively heterosexual orientation seems more likely on conceptual grounds; that is, given an innate, biological, heterosexual bias, and the fact that preferential homosexuality appears rooted in dysfunctional socialization. Such a change has been documented as a consequence of intensive psychoanalytic therapy (7). In a previous report, Pattison and Pattison (8) collated the small nonanalytic literature which documents such change, and they added 11 cases, eight of whom appeared to have achieved a successful and stable change.

Since the publication of that report, we have received an abundance of unsolicited personal accounts of such change. For example:

> A 30-year-old white male was a practicing exclusive homosexual for 10 years and a leader in the Gay community of a large city. He experienced a two-to-three-year transitional period to heterosexuality. He has a five-year, stable, happy marriage, and is a professional graduate student.

Another vignette is provided by a fellow psychiatrist:

> A 38-year-old white male, employed in a successful managerial position, considered himself an exclusive homosexual for many years. He had "overcome" his homosexuality with the assistance of a Christian Science practitioner. He did not engage in physical sexual relations with women, but he enjoyed women and reported active sexual fantasies about women. He reported he no longer had any sexual impulses toward males.

A philosophical self-help group, Aesthetic Realism, claims that several hundred of their members have changed from exclusively homosexual to exclusively heterosexual orientation (9).

As noted earlier, the largest and most-active proponent of

change in sexual orientation is a self-help movement, generally labelled the ex-Gay ministries. This movement has spawned indigenous small self-help groups, most affiliated with Protestant or Catholic church sponsorship. Although each is independent, there is a loose affiliative network, and national conferences. Such groups exist in at least 30 U.S. cities, as well as in England, France, Africa, Brazil, Australia, and elsewhere.

The commonality among the ex-Gay self-help programs is a religious ideology, offered as an alternative to Gay-liberation ideology. In brief, the Gay life style is defined as deviant; members are expected to participate in a "straight" life style. Homosexual orientation is defined as a developmental arrest; members are guided in psychosocial maturation. Sexual activity outside a monogamous, heterosexual marriage is defined as sinful; members are told they should live a sexually celibate life until or unless they can successfully enter a heterosexual marital and family life.

Participants in the ex-Gay movement offer a propitious natural experiment to study change in sexual orientation. Our first study was limited to just males, and from one program (8). In this Chapter we report results from a multiprogram survey, including both males and females.

METHOD

The survey questionnaire developed by Pattison and Pattison (8) was modified for self-administration, and field-tested for clarity. Agreements for program participation were arranged by Ms. Durrance. One hundred questionnaires were distributed to 20 ex-Gay programs in 11 states, whose program directors had agreed to identify long-term participants. Each subject completed the anonymous, self-administered questionnaire, which was returned by mail to Ms. Durrance. The questionnaire included open-ended completion items pertinent to past and present sexual history; sexual fantasies, dreams, and impulses; social relations; homosexual and heterosexual behavior and experiences; marital experience; details of alleged change in sexual orientation; participation in formal psychotherapy; and self-help group experience.

Table 1. Self-Report by 15 Subjects on Change in Sexual Orientation

Case	Gender	Age	Socio-economic Status*	Age at Homosexual Identification (Years)	Age of Change to Heterosexuality (Years)	Years as Exclusive Homosexual Orientation	Heterosexual Orientation	Marriage Data			Intrapsychic Evidence of Homosexuality	Kinsey Ratings	
								Age at Marriage (Years)	Years Married	Marital Happiness		Before Change	After Change
1	F	27	3	15	24	9	3	24	3	+	±	6	1
2	F	32	2	15	25	10	7	26	6	++	0	6	0
3	F	32	2	24	29	5	3	—	—	—	0	6	0
4	F	26	2	14	23	9	3	—	—	—	±	6	1
5	F	29	2	20	28	8	1	—	—	—	±	6	1
6	F	22	3	19	21	2	1	divorced	1	—	±	6	1
7	F	28	2	18	27	9	1	divorced	3	—	0	6	0
8	F	31	2	8	17	9	14	28	3	++	0	6	0
9	F	36	2	21	26	5	7	26	10	++	0	4	0
10	F	26	2	21	22	1	2	—	—	—	0	5	0
11	M	27	2	10	24	4	3	25	2	++	±	6	1
12	M	27	3	8	25	17	2	26	1	++	±	5	1
13	M	28	2	6	18	12	10	20	8	++	±	6	1
14	M	28	3	13	19	6	4	20	8	++	±	6	1
15	M	26	2	12	21	9	4	20	6	++	±	6	2

* Hollingshead–Redlich five-point scale

RESULTS

Individual and group data are presented, and compared with the data from the prior Pattison and Pattison study (8) (referred to as P and P hereafter).

Of 100 questionnaires, over 50 were returned with complete detail. The returns came from programs representing rural and urban settings, and diverse religious affiliations.

A preliminary review differentiated between "successful" program participation and change in sexual orientation. Two-thirds of our successful respondents were indeed successful program participants, but had not achieved a change in psychic sexual orientation. They described themselves as celibate homosexuals or as "learning to live straight." They were successful in the sense of pursuing the ideological life-style goals of the movement; but they were also frank in the admission of continued homosexual orientation in terms of psychological preference. We were left with less than one-third ($N = 15$) of our sample who claimed change in sexual orientation.

Sample Characteristics

As shown in Table 1, our sample consists of 15 white adults, 10 women and five men, between the ages of 27 and 36 years (mean age = 28 years). In terms of education and socioeconomic status, four subjects (two males, two females) had high-school educations and hold blue-collar jobs; the other 11 subjects had some college education and hold white-collar jobs. These age, education, and socioeconomic characteristics are almost identical to the P and P sample.

The age at which the subjects identified themselves as homosexual ranged from eight to 24 years (mean age = 15). This is the same mean age as the P and P sample, and compares well with other studies cited by P and P, that homosexual self-identification typically occurs in young adolescence. However, this sample included four women who did not identify as homosexual until age 20–24. This finding is consonant with the Kinsey Institute study

(1), which found that women may identify themselves as homosexual somewhat later in development.

Age at which the subjects identified change to heterosexual
orientation ranged from 17–29 years (mean age = 23). The number of years of exclusively homosexual identification and explicit
homosexual activity ranged from 1–14 years (mean = 8 years).
The number of years of exclusively heterosexual identification
ranged from 1–14 years (mean = 8 years). The means for each of
the above are identical to the mean figures in the P and P sample.
Similarly, Troiden (10) has reported that change in sexual orientation typically occurs in the 20–25-year-old period.

Kinsey Scale

We assessed the degree of sexual orientation on the Kinsey scale
(11). On a seven-point scale, a rating of zero is defined as exclusively heterosexual, while a rating of six is exclusively homosexual. A rating of one occurs with incidental psychic response to the
same gender.

In our sample the before–after scores on the Kinsey scale were:
6–0 (N = four); 6–1 (N = seven); 6–2 (N = one); 4–0 (N = one);
5–0 (N = one); 5–1 (N =one). Thus, in this sample, 14 of 15
subjects changed to a 0 or 1 level of exclusively heterosexual
orientation. In the P and P sample, eight of 11 subjects exhibited
such change.

Again, we were interested in evidence of lingering psychic
homosexual response that might be manifest in dreams, fantasy,
or impulse. In this sample we found five subjects with no intrapsychic evidence, nine subjects with incidental evidence, and one
subject with conflictual intrapsychic homosexual response. In the
prior P and P sample, three subjects had no intrapsychic evidence,
five had incidental evidence, and three subjects had manifest
intrapsychic response.

Heterosexual Marital Experience

In this sample, eight subjects are currently married (four out of
10 females, four out of five males). All reported high satisfaction

and marital happiness, except for one subject, who reported some marital conflict (subject number one). One subject (number 15) reported high marital satisfaction despite intrapsychic conflict. Two divorced women had been unhappily married during their actively homosexual periods. Of the unmarried, all are active in heterosexual dating. The age of marriage ranged from 20–28 years (mean age = 25). Years married ranged from 1–10 years (men = five years). In the P and P sample, the mean age at marriage was 24 years, and mean years married was four years. The satisfaction and successful marital pattern reported here is similar to the P and P sample, where there were six of 11 married, with one married subject with intrapsychic homosexual response.

Change, Maintenance, and "Cure"

The concept of *cure* has acquired negative ideological connotations, in that it implies a prior pathological or sick status to homosexual orientation. A less ideologically charged concept is that of *change*, particularly since we do not have much information on the stability, maintenance, or shift of sexual orientation over time on our subjects.

With the above caveat, we have used the Saghir and Robins (12) criteria for change:

> Thus a "cured" homosexual would not only disengage from homosexual activity but he would also disengage emotionally and to a large extent from homosexual attachments, including homosexual fantasies, dreams, and physical arousal by sight and touch (p. 319).

Accordingly, we conclude that the criteria for stable and nonconflictual change are met by six married subjects (four females, two males); that three dating subjects (two females, one male) probably meet the criteria; that five subjects (four females, one male) are equivocal, due to less than two years as heterosexual; and one subject, happily married, has intrapsychic conflict.

Nevertheless, we do not feel that our two small studies have adequately addressed the issue of stability and maintenance of change. We conducted an informal information survey in 1984 of the 11 subjects reported by P and P in 1980, a six-year follow-up period. Our sketchy information revealed that some subjects had changed back to homosexual orientation, some remain stably heterosexual, some fluctuate. This information (albeit inadequate), indicates that we *cannot assume* that once a person has become an exclusive heterosexual that such change is necessarily permanent. As Gadpaille (2) has emphasized, simple global ratings of sexual orientation, or even current behavioral data, do not provide an adequate assessment of the *qualitative* aspects of sexual orientation. Thus, among our nine subjects (six females, three males) who currently manifest stable, exclusively heterosexual orientation, there may well be significant prognostic differences in their intrapsychic organization of sexual orientation.

Further, we report that a number of our current survey respondents (nonchanged) expressed doubt about the concept of cure, and made a direct analogy to Alcoholics Anonymous. That is, they saw themselves as achieving a stable, nonhomosexual life style, but questioned their own capacity to totally change their psychic sexual orientation.

The problem of qualitative assessment of psychosexual orientation is further illustrated by the similarities and contrasts between our two sample groups. In our total sample of over 50 subjects, all had been active members and participants in the ex-Gay movement for at least two years. All shared the same religious ideology, similar group socialization, and similar behavioral reinforcements. All were living a "straight," non-Gay life style. Yet only a minority demonstrated a change in psychic psychosexual orientation. There were no significant differences between the unchanged and changed groups in terms of the descriptive data we have gathered (that is, age of homosexual identification, years as homosexual, attempts at heterosexuality, years of participation in the ex-Gay movement). Thus the psychosocial "change factors" of the ex-Gay movement may be necessary but not sufficient causes to change psychosexual orientation. At the same time, the maintenance of change in psychosexual orientation may be linked to continued reinforcement by group participation.

The parallel to alcoholism and Alcoholics Anonymous may be pertinent. In that case, not all alcoholics attain sobriety, even though they actively participate in AA; and the maintenance of sobriety appears to be strongly linked to continued participation in AA. (It is noteworthy that "spontaneous cures" also occur among alcoholics, and that some persons successfully leave AA after some years because they do not need that group reinforcement.)

Subject Perceptions of the Change Process

The themes of these responses are markedly similar, which no doubt reflects their acceptance and adherence to the ideology of the ex-Gay movement.

First, subjects described the sense of isolation, loneliness, and differentness from others. Although active in a Gay life style, they reported the continued internal sense of isolation from others as "different." Socialization and social acceptance in Gay community life did not redress the internal loneliness.

I felt so alone, so unlike others, I knew inside myself I was different.

The lie that homosexuality is a valid, happy life style is the most destructive . . . used to convince those involved that they are happy. It is my pleasure to share that joy and peace of living a life style free and in harmony . . .

This observation is consonant with the Kinsey Institute study (1), which reports that in latency, the homosexually oriented child experiences self as different and apart from peers. Similarly, Van den Aardweg (13) reported a study of childhood in 200 homosexuals, in which a primary experience of differentness and inferiority of self led to adult experiences of internal loneliness, self-pity, and self-depreciation. He notes that social acceptance in a Gay life style does not allay the internal loneliness of being different and unacceptable.

Second, there was a universal recognition that homosexual orientation involved more than just sexual attraction; that one's homosexual orientation reflected major maturational deficits in the affective and cognitive ego systems.

You cannot concentrate on becoming heterosexual, but rather, you must concentrate on becoming a whole person. There are so many other things to work on—homosexuality (you find out after a whole lotta hell) is just one part of the picture.

I was taught that the only way you can show love to someone is to have a physical relationship . . . I forgot what pure love meant . . . and even how it felt.

In my Gay experience, I depended totally on feelings—my emotions ruled my life . . . I've learned to say no to my feelings and yes to my commitments . . . I've followed through.

I couldn't even tell if a woman was pretty or not. Sitting and talking to a woman was like talking to a chair. The personalities of women were kind of out of focus, but the more I reached out in faith to them, the more that focus sharpened, and their different personalities became distinguished and attractive.

These themes, of course, are consonant with the general psycho-analytic view that homosexual orientation is more than a sexual preference, that it is a conflictual manifestation of impaired self-identity and object-relation maturation (14).

Third, the subjects noted that their change in sexual orientation had not been dramatic or magical, but rather was a long, tough road in personal growth. They emphasized the importance of accepting responsibility for one's life and making deliberate choices about one's actions. All the subjects had received some type of short-term religious counselling—although not intensive psychotherapy. But they placed primary emphasis on the importance of the self-help peer-group counselling.

Having close ex-Gay and Christian friends to counsel me at my speed, not theirs, was the difference.

I found out that homosexuality is a learned behavior . . . you're not born that way . . . and it has to be unlearned.

I had to learn to accept the truth and act upon it.

I had to learn to be honest—with God, self, and others.

Self-condemnation had to be replaced by self-acceptance.

Yes, homosexual desires are brought on by an unfulfilled emotional need. But because beliefs and thinking affect emotions, mental imbed-ding of the idea "I'm Gay, a faggot, queer, fairy" results in stronger homosexual emotions. The more there is indulgence in the homosex-ual act, the more the body becomes acclimated, habituated to that type of release. Increasingly there is that association between the same sex and perverted pleasure. The wrong thinking, the learned habit pattern are strong influences. One needs models. People who can say, "I really understand. Yes, I've been there, I've felt and thought the same as you. But change is possible. I've been set free."

The above quotations reflect the same genre of therapeutic ele-ments in *folk-healing*," described previously in P and P. Two recent books on self-help therapy (15, 16) are consonant with the processes described here: a group commitment to an ideology, a set of behavioral expectations, group acceptance, group guidance in experiential learning, and group support for living a new life style.

DISCUSSION

There are obvious methodological limitations in a study such as this. Self-report data are subject to reporter bias, especially in an area fraught with ideological conflict. However, two-thirds of our original survey sample did *not* report a change to exclusively heterosexual orientation; while the 15 subjects reported here pro-vided significant variations in their life histories, not all of one piece. Further, there is striking veridicality in this sample from different geographic programs with the data reported in our P & P sample. Thus there appears to be reasonable face validity to the data. A large national sample, based on personal interviews, is needed to ascertain validity and generalizability.

An important issue raised in our two studies is that of *mainte-nance of change*. Are the reported changes to exclusive heterosex-uality stable and permanent? Although we report stable exclu-sively heterosexual orientation for up to 14 years, it still remains to conduct longitudinal follow-up studies. Our informal follow-up information highlights the need for qualitative assessment, for it would appear that change to exclusive heterosexuality is stable and permanent in some, while quite unstable in others.

A third issue is the prediction of change in sexual orientation. Persons of bisexual orientation (Kinsey 3, 4) may change to exclusive heterosexuality. However, in our two studies we have focused on persons of exclusively homosexual orientation (Kinsey 5, 6). What predicts capacity for change and/or stability of change? Gadpaille (2) recommends the development of *qualitative* profiles that would contain such predictive variables.

Finally, we reiterate that these cases exemplify the fact that change in sexual orientation is anything but "natural" or "spontaneous." All of the cases reported here are the product of considerable therapy, in this case the process of participation in a religious self-help-group movement. In light of the accumulating sociocultural data, it would appear that social process and acculturation norms may play a more powerful role in the determination of ongoing sexual orientation than we have previously thought. In fact, sociocultural ideologies, usually embedded in religious belief, ritual, and social norming, may override intrapsychic processes per se. Yet intrapsychic elements of psychosexual orientation are still manifestly important and, as our samples illustrate, may not be easily influenced by psychosocial factors.

CONCLUSIONS

This study provides confirmatory data on change in sexual orientation from exclusive homosexuality to exclusive heterosexuality. The sample includes data on female subjects, and subjects from multiple sites. These data support our prior analysis of the relevance of a folk-healing process, in this case the ex-Gay self-help movement. Important elements in producing change include ideology, behavioral expectations, and behavioral experience. Our evidence again suggests that cognitive change occurs first, followed by behavioral change, and finally intrapsychic change. However, the *maintenance* of change in sexual orientation is open to question. Qualitative aspects of sexual orientation need to be specified in longitudinal research, instead of global ratings of sexual orientation. Accumulating sociocultural evidence suggests that social and cultural norms and expectations, typically embedded in religious ideology, may play a major role in the development, maintenance, or change of sexual orientation. In sum, our data and reflections thereon suggest further reconsideration of what constitutes human psychosexual orientation.

Psychosexual Orientation in Anthropology

We have already alluded to the concept of socialization into gender-dimorphic roles. That is, society establishes and socializes persons into dichotomized male and female gender roles, which are also sexual roles, or vice versa. It has been assumed in most psychodynamic theory that a homosexual orientation results from a failure of such appropriate socialization within the family of rearing.

This view has been challenged by a substantive body of current anthropological research in Melanesia, where a majority of societies practice universal ritualized homosexuality among males, as part of socialization into manhood. Thus, although all males go through a period of religiously ritualized homosexual behavior, almost all males then proceed to the next step of masculinization, where they marry, bear children, and remain monogamous, heterosexual husbands and fathers. Of note is the fact that such universal ritualized homosexuality is not associated with the effeminacy, cross-gender behavior, or other sexual "deviance" that Western societies identify with homosexuality (17, 18).

This data suggests that family dynamics, per se, may not be a critical nexus for the development of gender orientation, but rather the larger sociocultural milieu of gender/role socialization is implicated. Thus, sexual behavior, per se, may not be indicative of or predictive of psychosexual preferential orientation. The Melanesian data suggest that, at least for males, the socialization process from the beginning is gender-dimorphic. The route to becoming a heterosexual male includes a period of sexual behavior as a homosexual male. Thus, sexual behavior is a consequence rather than a cause. Sexual preference and orientation seem embedded in more profound aspects of psychosexual identity.

This proposition is further explicated in the work of Ortner and

Whitehead (19). They examine the cultural construction of gender and sexuality in a variety of non-Western societies, including
both male and female perspectives. In brief, they distinguish between homosexual sexual acts, homosexual appearance (dressing
in the role of the opposite gender), and homosexual social role
(working in the role of the opposite gender). In their ethnographic
analyses, it is of interest that psychosexual orientation is primarily
expressed in social appearance and social vocational activities.
That is, heterosexual orientation is expressed via clear, gender-
dimorphic role attributes which are socially visible. On the other
hand, homosexual sexual behavior, per se, appears much less
significant. In such societies, a homosexual psychosexual orientation is expressed in gender identification and gender role attribu-
tion. Only incidentally does homosexual genital sexual behavior
play a role. Consequently, homosexual contact is not defined as
the primary definer of sexuality. The heterosexual may have
occasional, ceremonial, or incidental genital homosexual contacts,
which are not perceived as pertaining to psychosexual identity or
psychosexual orientation. All of this stands in contrast to the
current Western milieu, where gender and gender roles have been
substantially dissociated from social dress, social behavior, and
social vocational roles. As a consequence, the only major
"marker" of gender identity is that of sexual contact! Such may be
an underlying cultural reason for the current Western preoccupa-
tion with displays of genital sexuality in public media—How else
to distinguish men from women? At the same time, homosexual
orientation has come to be psychodynamically defined in terms of
genital sexual preference, replacing the understanding of psychosexual orientation as part of a fundamental, dimorphic differentiation of identity between men and women.

These anthropological lines of research in many ways support
the more traditional psychoanalytic formulations of homosexuality as an expression of gender identity. At the same time, this
research radically challenges the notion of gender identity as
rooted in sexuality. Perhaps it is quite the other way around:
Sexuality is rooted in gender identity.

This whole line of investigation leads back to religion, for

religious systems typically formulate powerful sociocultural definitions of masculinity and femininity, male and female. In some
religions, the masculine and the feminine are always found
within each gender; in others the masculine and the feminine are
opposed and in perpetual tension; while in still others, the masculine and the feminine unite to create a unitary human. Further, in
traditional societies and cultures, there is a fusion of religion and
culture, such that they cannot be separated. Thus, the cultural
pattern of dimorphic gender socialization is a religious process, and
vice versa. It is intriguing to speculate whether the ex-Gay movement that we have been studying may be an example of a subcultural phenomenon of religion–culture, which has an inherent
socialization process promoting gender differentiation, and which
consequently modifies the psychosexual orientation of its mem-
bership.

Ideology: Gay Liberation versus Ex-Gay

The lines of research reported here have understandably pro-
voked strong ideological reactions. The Gay-liberation movement
has taken the ideological position that homosexual orientation is
immutable and, even if change is possible, it is unnecessary and/or
undesirable. For example, recent Gay-liberation spokespersons
have vigorously criticized clinical and research work on change in
sexual orientation, as well as attacking the ideological stance of the
ex-Gay movement (20). In turn, the ex-Gay movement has been
perhaps unrealistically enthusiastic about any evidence of change
in homosexual orientation, and has been likewise critical of the
ideological propositions of the Gay-liberation movement.

What is lacking in such ideological debates is a clear appreciation for the complexity of what we glibly term sexuality. As we
have tried to set forth in this work, sexuality is linked to gender, to
roles, to beliefs, and to values. It would be impossible to understand the research data discussed here without an appreciation for
the functions of ideology in the construction of social realities.
And, in large part, religious ideology plays a central role in most
cultural constructions of reality. Thus, it is part of the research

agenda to investigate how religious ideologies relate to the operation of human sexuality. We do not believe it possible to accurately apprehend the development, maintenance, or change of psychosocial orientation purely as biological phenomena, since the evidence appears so suasive that human sexuality is a biopsychosocial behavior. Thus we would not exclude biological determinants, although they are not discussed here. Rather, we have sought to explicate the relatively neglected sociocultural components of human sexuality, which for most cultures is thereby also a religious component.

SUMMARY

We report here further survey evidence of change in homosexual orientation to heterosexual orientation in a subcultural religious population. Our findings have led to a consideration of pertinent recent anthropological research that demonstrates how sociocultural constructions of gender, identity, and sexuality play a critical role in psychosexual orientation. Such ethnographic data also demonstrate how dimorphic gender socialization is typically embedded in religious frameworks. Thus our research on a religious subculture appears consonant with parallel ethnographic data. Finally, since human sexuality is defined and given meaning by sociocultural constructions of reality, we are inevitably led to competing social ideological formulations. In the case at hand in our own culture, we see the Gay-liberation movement struggling with the ex-Gay movement to achieve opposing social and religious meanings of sexuality.

References

1. Bell AP, Weinberg MS, Hammersmith SK: Sexual Preference: Its Development in Men and Women. Bloomington, Indiana University Press, 1981

2. Gadpaille WJ: Cross-species and cross-cultural contributions to understanding homosexual activity. Arch Gen Psychiatry 37:349–356, 1980

3. Herdt GH: Guardians of the Flutes: Idioms of Masculinity. New York, McGraw-Hill, 1980

4. Bryant C: Sexual Deviancy and Social Proscription. New York, Human Sciences Press, 1982

5. Bullough VL: Sexual Variance in Society and History. Chicago, University of Chicago Press, 1980

6. Altshuler KZ: On the question of bisexuality. Am J Psychother 38:484–493, 1984

7. Socarides CW: Homosexuality. New York, Jason Aronson, 1978

8. Pattison EM, Pattison ML: Ex-Gays: religiously mediated change in homosexuals. Am J Psychiatry 137:1553–1562, 1980

9. Kranz S: The H Persuasion. New York, Definition Press, 1981

10. Troiden RR: Becoming homosexual: a model of gay identity acquisition. Psychiatry 42:362–372, 1979

11. Kinsey A, Pomeroy W, Martin C: Sexual Behavior in the Human Male. Philadelphia, WB Saunders Co, 1948

12. Saghir MT, Robins E: Male and Female Homosexuality. Baltimore, Williams & Wilkins, 1973

13. Van den Aardweg GJM: Parents of homosexuals—not guilty? interpretation of childhood psychological data. Am J Psychother 38:180–189, 1984

14. Nelson MC, Ikenberry J: Psychosexual Imperatives: Their Role in Identity Formation. New York, Human Sciences Press, 1979

15. Weber GH, Cohen LM: Beliefs and Self-Help: Cross-Cultural Perspectives and Approaches. New York, Human Sciences Press, 1982

16. Katz AH, Bender EI: The Strength in Us: Self-Help Groups in the Modern World. New York, New Viewpoints Press, 1976

17. Herdt GM: Rituals of Manhood. Berkeley, University of California Press, 1982

18. Herdt GM: Ritualized Homosexuality in Melanesia. Berkeley, University of California Press, 1984

19. Ortner SB, Whitehead M: Sexual Meanings: The Cultural Construction of Gender and Sexuality. New York, Cambridge University Press, 1981

20. Martin AD: The emperor's new clothes: modern attempts to change sexual orientation, in Psychotherapy with Homosexuals. Edited by Hetrick ES, Stein TS. Washington DC, American Psychiatric Press, Inc., 1984

10

The Measurement of Religion in Psychiatric Research

David B. Larson, M.D., M.S.P.H.
E. Mansell Pattison, M.D.
Dan G. Blazer, M.D., Ph.D.
Abdul R. Omran, M.D., D.P.H.
Berton H. Kaplan, Ph.D.

10

The Measurement of
Religion in
Psychiatric Research

In the last 10 years four national surveys (1–4) have documented the highly religious orientation of the United States population. Extracting from these surveys, over 90 percent of the population believe in God, over 35 percent attend church on a weekly basis or with greater frequency, and over 20 percent perceive religion to be "very important" to them.

In contrast, Ragan et al. (5), reporting on a large sample of members of the American Psychological Association, found that only five percent believed in God. In a study including most of the members of the American Psychiatric Association (6), some 43 percent believed in God. The other 57 percent had either agnostic or atheistic beliefs. Turning to religious practices, Henry et al., in their analyses of mental health professionals from Chicago, Los Angeles, and New York (7), found that 15 percent of those sampled practiced their religions on a regular basis. The other 85 percent practiced their religions on a "light" or "none" basis. On the other hand, assessing those of the Protestant, Roman Catholic, or Jewish faiths, the American Psychiatric Association Task Force Report No. 10 (6) found some 27 percent went to church or

---

The views expressed in this chapter are those of the authors, and no official endorsement by NIMH is intended or should be inferred.

synagogue on a regular basis, with the other 73 percent attending "occasionally" to "never."

The study by Henry and colleagues (7) also evaluated the proportion of mental health professionals who came from theistic homes but were no longer theistic themselves. Of the 3,286 who came from theistic homes, 928 or 28 percent no longer maintained these theistic beliefs. This 28 percent reduction is huge when compared to the change in theistic beliefs found between two generations in the general population. From 1944 to 1981, the Gallup Poll interviewed Americans a dozen times about their belief in God (4). In 1944, 96 percent believed in God; in 1981, 95 percent believed in God. The mean for the 12 surveys was 96.25 percent, with a very small standard error of 0.49 percent. We cannot say if this large intergenerational religious change is unique to mental health professionals. It would be important to assess other groups of professionals to see if a similarly extensive intergenerational change occurs.

It is one thing to suggest that mental health professionals have differing religious views or religious commitments than do the general public; it is another to show that mental health professionals and their patients do have divergent religious views or values. There is a small literature that has documented such findings. Lillienfeld (8) found large differences between therapists' values and their mostly Roman Catholic clientele's. Vaughn's study (9) had similar findings. Although clinical theory espouses a lack of value orientation, many authors (10–16) have discussed the presence of value-laden views among mental health professionals. Research needs to be done to further assess not only the presence of therapist–patient value differences, but also their impact on psychotherapy outcomes.

Given these findings, we have sought to evaluate the extent to which psychiatric research acknowledges and assesses the role of religion in the lives of psychiatric patients. We undertook a systematic review of the most representative psychiatric literature, assessing the relevance of religious measures in terms of quantity and quality of religious variables used. For quantity, the frequency of the number of religious variables per total studies is calculated.

For quality of the research, several aspects will be analyzed: 1) the measures' usefulness; 2) the extent to which the authors referenced the available religious literature; and 3) the comparability to other recent reviews of religious research in the psychosocial literature.

DENOMINATION AND RELIGIOSITY MEASURES

Many might be familiar with the Protestant–Roman Catholic differences that Durkheim (17) found for suicide. This early sociological tradition of assessing differences between denominations was particularly encouraged by Niebuhr in his 1929 book, *Social Sources of Denominationalism.* More recently, Harrison and Lazerwitz (18) have noted factors that blur denominational differences between Protestant and Catholic groups. Roof (19) has written about the emergence of many Protestant religious groups, quite different in ethnic, racial, and cultural backgrounds. Wuthnow (20) has discussed the erosion of religious traditionalism within the denominations. Hoge (21) and Etheridge and Feagin (22) have found a diverse range of religious styles among individuals of the same denomination. As a result of the above findings, one would not expect the quantification of religious denominations to be a useful research variable.

We will now turn our attention to more dynamic religious measures. Kaufman (23), acknowledging Finner (24) and Himmelfarb (25), has defined the more dynamic measure of religiosity as, "The degree to which religious beliefs, attitudes, and behaviors permeate the life of an individual" (p. 237). Religiosity is seen to consist of a number of aspects or dimensions (such as religious practices, beliefs, and attitudes); thus, multidimensional religious scales measuring a combination of religious dimensions have been created. Moberg (26) argues for the value and importance of using multidimensional religiosity items and not single, unidimensional religious questions. Hadaway (27) has written that these scales or questions should be at least composed of religious-meaning (for example, frequency of prayer) and belonging (for example, frequency of attendance) items. Pattison (28) has described religion as a complex phenomenon, multivariate in form and function: "No one religious factor operates in isolation, but in (various) permutations and combinations of multiple religious factors" (28, p. 114). Roof (29) would agree with Pattison and Moberg; he proposed that religious commitment needs to be assessed multidimensionally—whether using a single multidimensional scale or several questions, each unidimensional in form. Gorsuch (30) emphasizes that whatever form of scale is used should be dependent on both the underlying theory and the particular questions being asked.

Glock and Stark (31) have developed the most widely known religiosity measure. They proposed five dimensions:

1. *Ideological:* Referring to commitment to a group or movement as a social process

2. *Intellectual:* Referring to a specific set of beliefs, explanations, or cognitive structuring of meaning and value

3. *Experiential:* Referring to the feelings one experiences, which may be entirely personal, or may result from structured group activities producing specific experiences

4. *Sacramental:* Referring to participation in symbolic rituals

5. *Consequential:* Referring to religiously defined standards of conduct

As noted by Kaufman, "most investigators accept the validity of the belief, ritual, devotional, and experience dimensions and have produced data which empirically support such (dimensions)" (23, p. 239). There has not been as much support for either the intellectual or consequential dimensions.

CITATION OF THE AVAILABLE RELIGIOUS LITERATURE

Carolyn Mullins has written that the behavioral scientist needs to reference resources used in order to "acknowledge all intellectual debts [and] document all facts and ideas that are not common knowledge or not original with [the author]" (32, pp. 41–42).

These concepts are further supported in Warriner's *English Grammar and Composition* (33). Our study investigates how well the authors of the studies that include religious variables did (or did not) acknowledge their debts (or assumed the religious variable to be common knowledge in the form used). Expectations are that if the religious research is of high quality, the available religious literature will be frequently cited. If the religious research is of low quality, the available literature will be infrequently cited. In addition, we expected that the more resources referenced, the greater will be the proportion of religiosity (versus denomination) questions asked. On the other hand, if few or no resources were cited, a greater proportion of denomination (versus religiosity) questions would be asked.

RECENT REVIEWS OF RELIGION IN PSYCHIATRY, SOCIOLOGY, AND PSYCHOLOGY

There has been one recent review of religion and mental health in the psychiatric literature, published by Sanua (34) in 1969. This study reviewed a variety of empirical studies to evaluate whether "religion is a basis of sound mental health, general well-being, and humanitarianism." This was not a review of the psychiatric literature pertaining to research methods; rather, it was a review of such sociological and psychological literature as might answer the question. Of the 67 references, only one was from the psychiatric literature; that came from the *Guild of Catholic Psychiatrists Bulletin*. This journal is not widely circulated or cited.

With respect to the recommendations made by Light and Pillemer (35), there were the following problems with the Sanua review. First, there was no sampling frame or procedure to determine 1) which journals were reviewed; 2) which studies were excluded; 3) how many total studies were assessed; 4) what proportion of all the studies included religious measures; and 5) what types of religious measures were quantified. Without an objective, clear, criteria-based frame, it is not only difficult to replicate the review, but selection bases affecting which studies are chosen can become uncontrolled. In addition, there was no quantification of the data as they related to the original hypothesis. That is, it was not specified which studies showed significant associations between 1) religion and mental health; 2) religion and mental illness; 3) both 1 and 2; or 4) neither 1 nor 2. Without quantified results we wonder how the author was able to answer his original question—much less, make conclusions about his findings.

Buehler et al. (36) systematically reviewed how religious variables were researched in the four major American sociological journals for the 1890–1969 time period. During the 80 years investigated, five percent of all of the journal research articles included religious variables. Two-thirds of the quantitative studies assessing religion used descriptive statistics (that is, means, modes, ranges, and so forth), contrasting with the other third using inferential test statistics (that is, χ^2 test, t test z test, and the like). Of the total number of religious dependent and independent variables used, 23.3 percent used religiosity measures, while 10.6 percent used denomination. Thus the religiosity-to-denominational ratio was 2.2:1. This is a rather surprising result, since religion, measured multidimensionally, did not come into the forefront of the sociological literature until Lenski's (37) concept of "religious interests."

Capps et al. (38), in a less-systematic but more-extensive review of some 50 journals from the fields of sociology, psychology, and religion, found 1,869 articles relevant to the psychology of religion during a recent 25-year period (1950–1974). Unlike Buehler et al., this study did not include the total number of articles reviewed from the 50 journals. Thus one cannot estimate the proportion of all studies that measured the psychology of religion. One can estimate the percentage of the 1,869 articles with either religiosity or denominational variables. The ratio of religiosity to denominational variables in this literature was 3:1, greater than the ratio for the sociological review. This difference should not be that surprising, since historically sociology has been more concerned with class measures (like denomination), while psychology has been more concerned with dynamic measures (such as religiosity). Also, the Capps et al. review was for 1950–1974, whereas the Buehler et al. review was for 1890–1969. The latter review included earlier years of the twentieth century, when denomination was used more extensively in differentiating social or cultural factors.

METHOD

In order to obtain the most-recent and -representative sample of the highest quality English-language psychiatric research, the American, British, and Canadian Journals of Psychiatry along with the *Archives of General Psychiatry* were reviewed for the 1978–1982 time period. All 3,777 articles were evaluated for at least one religious variable which was quantified, using either descriptive or inferential statistics. Consistent with the methods of Buehler et al. (36), only quantified research was included. Thus, case reports and theoretical or review papers were excluded from those studies reviewed. Of a possible 3,777 articles from the four journals, there were 1,412 articles excluded due to their lack of quantification. An additional 17 studies were excluded, since they pertained to sects or cults. The authors felt that the forms that these religious beliefs take in a Western context are quite divergent from the forms that the Catholic, Jewish, and Protestant faiths take in the same context (39, 40). Thus, a total of 1,429 articles, or 37.8 percent of 3,777 articles, were excluded, leaving 2,348 studies to be assessed.

Evaluating the 2,348 quantified studies, there were 59 articles that both included a quantified religious variable and did not fit any of the exclusion criteria. A metric was considered to be a descriptive statistic if it was a "summary characteristic of a sample of observations" (41, p. 91). In this case, one could make interpretations about the results based on measures of central tendencies (for example, the mean or percentage of the total) or indicators of variability (for example, the standard deviation) (41). A metric was considered an inferential statistic if a test statistic (that is, z, t, f- tests) was used to evaluate and interpret the results (41). If the study contained both descriptive and inferential statistics analyzing religion, it was tabulated as an inferential study. If the study included both religious denomination and a religiosity measure, it was enumerated as a religiosity study. Thus, to be considered a denominational study, it could only contain a measure assessing one's religious denomination.

Statistical tests for the no-difference hypotheses were done using a two-sided χ^2 test statistic. The five statistical tests were done in the results from Tables 2, 7, and 8. The alpha level was set at .01 due to the exploratory nature of the research (42), using the Bonferroni method outlined in Kleinbaum and Kupper (43).

RESULTS

To begin with, about three-eighths of the studies in all four journals were excluded because they did not use either an inferential or a descriptive statistic. Of those that did, the *Archives of General Psychiatry* and the *British Journal of Psychiatry* had significantly greater frequencies of inferential statistics than did the *American Journal of Psychiatry* or the *Canadian Journal of Psychiatry*. For all four journals the inferential/descriptive ratio was 1,896:452, or about 4:1.

Table 1 addresses: Was the inferential/descriptive ratio of 4:1 found for the four journals for the five-year period similar to the ratio found for the 59 studies that included religious variables? As can be seen, it was not. The resulting ratio (38:21) of 1.80 is more than 50 percent less than the 4.2 level. Using a χ^2 test, the *p* value is < .01. Thus there is a difference in the proportion of studies using inferential (versus descriptive) statistics between the 59 studies that used religious variables and the 2,289 studies that did not.

Table 2 addresses: How frequently is at least one religious question included in the recent psychiatric research? The frequency rates were determined by using the data from all four journals for the denominator and the data from Table 2 for the numerator. Overall, one in 40 quantitative studies included at least one single religious question. If all studies where only a religiosity question was asked are included, the frequency rate decreased to one article in 107.

Unlike Tables 1 and 2, which presented data for all the four journals studies, Tables 3–5 analyze data for the religiosity and/or denominational questions included in the 59 studies only. Starting with Table 4, of the 59 studies, the great majority had a single religious question, with only 10 studies having two or more religious questions (that is, either denomination or religiosity measures).

Table 4 permits us to clarify: Of the 59 studies, 1) how many having a religious question assessed religiosity? and 2) how many had two or more religiosity questions? Concerning the first question, 22 (37 percent) of those studies with a religious question analyzed religiosity. The other 63 percent analyzed denomination alone. As to the second question, five (less than 10 percent of the total) had two or more religiosity questions. Thus, in the psychiatric literature between 1978 and 1982, one quantified study in about 400 had two or more religiosity questions.

In evaluating how frequently the authors of the 59 studies included a religious citation, we see in Table 5 that 51 studies did not have any religious references, two articles (three percent) had one reference, and six (10 percent) had two or more references. Given our prior discussion, it would be expected that the authors who referenced the religious literature had proportionately more

Table 1. Type of Religious Variable and Statistic Used

(Total = 59 studies)	Denomination	Religiosity	Inferential Statistic	Descriptive Statistic
American	10	8	8	10
Archives	13	8	16	5
British	5	4	6	3
Canadian	9	2	8	3
Totals	37	22	38	21

Table 2. Frequency Rates for the Use of at Least One Religious Question per All the Quantitative Studies

	Denomination	Religiosity	Total
American	1 in 91.4	1 in 114.25	1 in 51.8
Archives	1 in 48.5	1 in 78.75	1 in 30.0
British	1 in 127.4	1 in 159.25	1 in 70.8
Canadian	1 in 18.6	1 in 83.5	1 in 15.2
Totals	1 in 64.4	1 in 106.7	1 in 39.8

religiosity questions than the authors who did not reference the literature. Since there is a great amount of variation if two studies (42, 43) are included, we first analyzed the data in Table 6 for the 57 articles, excluding these two studies. Then we added them in, recalculating the results.

As expected, the greater the number of religious citations, the greater the number of religiosity (as opposed to denomination) questions asked. Likewise, the fewer the religious citations, the fewer the religiosity questions asked. Excluding references 42 and 43, the percentages of religiosity questions increased from 24 for

Table 3. Frequencies of Religious Questions Asked

Number of Religious Questions Asked per Study	Studies Assessed (2,348)	
	Number	Percentage
One	49	83.0
Two	8	13.6
Three or more	2	3.4
Total	59	100.0

Table 4. Frequencies of Religiosity and Denominational Questions Asked

Number of Religiosity and/or Denominational Question(s) Asked per Study	Studies Assessed (2,348)	
	Number	Percentage
One denominational question	37	63
One religiosity question	12	20
One denominational and one religiosity question	5	9
Two religiosity questions	3	5
Three or more religiosity questions	2	3
Total	59	100

Table 5. Frequencies of Religious Resources Referenced

Number of Religious Resources Referenced	Studies Assessed (2,348)	
	Number	Percentage
None	51	86.4
One	2	3.4
Two or more	6	10.2
Total	59	100.0

one question and no references, to 63 for the next level, to 83 for two or more questions and two or more references. The overall χ^2 p value for the 3×3 table, excluding 42 and 43, was $< .01$; including them, the χ^2 p value was $\leq .0001$.

Results shown in Table 7 enable us to evaluate two issues:

1. Did the number of psychiatric studies using denomination differ from the number of psychology or sociology studies using denomination?

2. Did the number of psychiatric studies using religiosity differ from the number of psychology or sociology studies using religiosity?

Starting with the first question, we see that the number of psychiatric studies assessing denomination was significantly more ($p < .01$) than sociology and significantly less ($p < .001$) than psychology. Thus, the frequency of psychiatry studies that as-

Table 6. The Distribution of the Studies Based on the Number of Religious Questions and the Number of Religious References

	5 Studies		8 Studies	46 Studies
	More than two religious references and more than two religious questions		One or more religious references and one religious question; OR no religious references and two or more religious questions	One religious question and no religious references
Percentage of questions— denomination	17 2	(1/6)* (1/50)**	37 (7/19)	76 (35/46)
Percentage of questions— denomination	83 98	(5/6)* (49/50)**	63 (12/19)	24 (11/46)
Totals (percent)	100* 100**		100	100

* Excludes references 42 and 43
** Includes references 42 and 43

sessed denomination was intermediate, although significantly different from either the sociology or psychology reviews.

Concerning the second question, psychiatry evaluated religiosity variables much less frequently than did either of the other psychosocial sciences. Both of the p values were less than .00005. These results are somewhat surprising, since the psychiatry review was much more recent than the other two reviews, thus one should have expected an even greater religiosity/denomination ratio than that found for the other two reviews. Yet the psychiatry ratio was less than one-fourth the sociology ratio and almost one-seventh the psychology ratio.

CONCLUSIONS

Our findings show that psychiatric research between 1978 and 1982:

1. infrequently included a quantified religious measure

2. very infrequently included a religiosity question

3. included a denomination measure at a greater frequency than it did religiosity measures

4. included single religiosity measures at a greater frequency than two or more (that is, "multiple") religiosity measures

Table 7. Comparison of the Religiosity and Denomination Use in Three Literature Reviews

Literature Reviews	Years Covered	Number of Studies Assessed	Number and Percentage of Studies Using Denomination	Number and Percentage of Studies Using Religiosity	Ratio of Religiosity to Denomination
Sociology	1890–1969	9,485	100 (1.0%)	219 (2.3%)	2.2
Psychology	1950–1974	1,869	66 (3.5%)	242 (12.9%)	3.7
Psychiatry	1978–1982	2,348	42 (1.8%)	22 (0.9%)	0.5

* 42 + 22 do not add up to 59 since five studies included both denomination and religiosity questions (see Table 4)

Reprinted from Larson D: Systematic analysis of research on religion in four major psychiatric journals: 1978–1982. Am J Psychiatry, March 1986. Reprinted by permission.

5. significantly and less frequently assessed religiosity than did either the comparable sociological or psychological literatures

6. infrequently cited the available sociological, psychological, and religious literature

Taking the first and second items above, of the 2,348 articles assessed, one religious question was found in every 40 articles. More importantly, less than one in 100 studies included a religiosity measure. It is surprising that less than one percent of the very recent psychiatric literature included a religious measure that might make a difference. It is particularly surprising given the proportions of the population that not only believe in God but are very committed to their religious faiths. In addition, it is even more surprising given the frequency with which mental health issues and religious dynamics overlap (41–65).

Considering the third item, 37 (63 percent) of the papers evaluated denomination, while 17 (28 percent) assessed religiosity. Five studies assessed both. Thus, over two times the number of studies that included measures of religiosity included denominational measures. This was unexpected. Actually, we expected the reverse to occur, with the frequency of studies using religiosity measures being far higher than those assessing denomination.

Turning to the fourth item, 17 (19 percent) of the 59 studies included a single religiosity variable. On the other hand, five studies (8 percent), a frequency more than three times the former, included two or more (that is, "multidimensional") religiosity variables. Like the second item, this result was again unexpected. We expected the reverse, with far more studies using multidimensional religiosity scales than single religious questions. In a review that is now more than three years out of date, Silverman (66) found 292 religious scales that would combine at least two questions to arrive at a numerical result. Although there were five studies in this review with two or more religious questions, only one (45) had used a scaled religious measure.

As to the fifth item, psychiatry assessed religiosity much less frequently than did either sociology or psychology. Thus, not only did psychiatry infrequently 1) look at religion at all and 2) measure several (or more) religiosity questions, but, when compared to other psychosocial reviews, it 3) very infrequently assessed religiosity. The questions that need to be asked are "Why does psychiatry so infrequently evaluate religion, and then, when it does, why does it do so at such a substandard level of quality?"

As to why these results occurred, several alternatives are possible. First, this particular set of results could be an unusual distribution of studies for the psychiatric literature. We were able to demonstrate a statistical difference in the descriptive/inferential distributions for the 59 studies including religious questions versus the other 2,289 studies. But we would need to go farther than this to document a "difference" in the populations of studies reviewed. We would need to show that either before and/or after this five-year period, the same four journals might have had, for example, significantly more religious questions, or more religiosity (consequently, less denominational) questions. Inter-time-review comparisons could then be made.

Secondly, our choice of journals could have been more biased than we originally expected. Thus, other psychiatric journals might have been more representative of the distribution of the various types of psychiatric research (for example, biological, psychotherapeutic, epidemiologic, social, and so forth) that we were hoping to have in the four journals selected. Or, for some reason, there was a bias against using religious measures in the four psychiatric journals selected. To assess these issues, a review of other psychiatric journals would need to be done for the same five years, demonstrating a different distribution of psychiatric research than that found in these four psychiatric journals. Or, another review would need to be done, demonstrating the decreased use of quantified religious questions and religiosity (as opposed to denomination) questions in this review.

A third explanation is the *small-study bias* described in Peto et al. (67). Most of the 59 studies included and analyzed had sample sizes of 30 or less; thus, there was an increased possibility for both type I errors, or false positives (67), and type II errors, or false negatives (68), to occur. To deal with the type I error, using a Bonferroni approach, we reset our alpha to .01. If the problem was of a type II nature, there would have been even more hypotheses rejected, substantiating the results of this paper even more so.

Two alternatives derive from the fifth and final item—the infrequently cited available sociological, psychological, and religious literature. As expected, the greater the number of religiosity questions, the greater the number of religious references cited. Thus one might conclude that psychiatric researchers made false assumptions both about the lack of the clinical usefulness of religiosity variables and about the greater usefulness of denominational (as opposed to religiosity) measures. As to the former assumption, research to be presented in a future paper will show that the religiosity hypotheses tested in these 59 studies had significant results (p value $< .05$) in over 50 percent of the statistical tests made.

The fifth and last alternative is that data were "dredged," referred to by David Sacket as *data-dredging bias* (69). Feinstein and Horowitz (70) have discussed *hypotheses-generating activities* where a "positive finding was presented as though it confirmed a preconceived hypothesis" (47, p. 1616). Thus there might have been data that looked as though it was tested on an a priori basis, when in reality, it was tested on an a posteriori bases. Various studies (43, 71) have shown how such statistical maneuvering resets the alpha to a much higher level than an assumed .05 level. Since only eight of the studies had referenced the literature at all, one wonders how the authors in the other 51 studies could conceive of their hypotheses on an a priori basis.

In summary, what should be done empirically in future psychiatric research concerning religion? First, religious measures should be included more frequently in psychiatric research. Little research has yet been done to analyze the interplay between religious and psychiatric dynamics. Steps need to be taken to evaluate this area far more frequently and more objectively. Secondly, if religion is to be clinically assessed, one should include religiosity measures, not denominational measures. Actually, one should include multidimensional religiosity measures with an acceptable reliability (26, 28, 30, and 72). Thirdly, one should include the religiosity measures that might be most affected by either the psychiatric status or the psychiatric intervention to be evaluated. The clinical–medical literature has already had enough studies that assess a single, superficial religious issue.

The lack of literature reviews shows that, at present, psychiatric researchers do not even consider the religious literature. Thus psychiatric research is a "leap of faith" away from the critical thinking needed to get us to a level of acceptable research (73–76). What should be done conceptually? The first step would be to review the literature in order to consider applicable sociological and/or psychological theoretical frameworks. The second step would then be to decide on the hypotheses about psychiatric–religious associations, or outcomes, to be tested. The third step would be to review the religious literature to choose a reliable multidimensional religiosity measure that would fit with the particular psychiatric dynamics or response (from an intervention) to be assessed. The fourth and final step is to undertake studies where reliable religious and psychiatric measures are included as dependent–independent variable (and vice versa) pairs. In addition, religious and psychiatric measures should be assessed both as independent variables with other clinically important outcome measures. The latter might include measures of social functioning, physical disease (for example, staging), and direct or indirect costs. With these steps we will start to make some scientific sense about how psychiatric dynamics and spiritual processes help, harm, hamper, or have "no effect" on each other.

In conclusion, although in 1965 both Pruyser (61) and Hiltner (62) were optimistic about the continuing dialogue of psychiatry and religion, we are not as enthusiastic about such synthesis 20 years later. There is a need for greater objectivity on both sides. Research provides just such a format for increased objectivity. Using a Kuhnian approach (73, 74), research should provide a means to move from the preparadigmatic, or polarized level, to the paradigmatic, or synthesizing stage. Our hope is that findings and recommendations like these might restart such progressive movement.

References

1. The Connecticut Mutual Life Report on American Values in the Eighties. Hartford, Connecticut Mutual Life Insurance Company, 1981

2. Veroff J, Douvan E, Kulka R: The Inner American. New York, Basic Books, 1981

3. Hadaway CK: Life satisfaction and religion: a re-analysis. Social Forces 57:636–643, 1978

4. Gallup G: Religion in America: 50 years, 1935–1985. Gallup Report 236, May 1985

5. Ragan CP, Malony NH, Beit-Hallahmi B: Psychologists and Religion: Professional Factors Related to Personal Religiosity. Paper presented at the Annual Meeting of the American Psychological Association, Washington, DC, September, 1976

6. Franzblau AN: Psychiatrists' Viewpoints on Religion and Their Services to Religious Institutions and the Ministry. Task Force Report No. 10. Washington, DC, American Psychiatric Association, 1975

7. Henry WE, Simms JH, Spray SL: The Fifth Profession: Becoming a Psychotherapist. San Francisco, Jossey-Bass 1971

8. Lillienfeld DM: The Relationship Between Mental Information and Moral Values of Lower Class Psychiatric Clinic Patients and Psychiatric Evaluation and Disposition. Doctoral dissertation, Columbia University, 1965. Dissertation Abstracts 27:610B–611B, 1966

9. Vaughn JL: Measurement and Analysis of Values Pertaining to Psychotherapy and Mental Health. Doctoral dissertation, Columbia University, 1971. Dissertation Abstracts 32:3655B–3656B, 1971

10. London P: The Modes and Morals of Psychotherapy. New York, Holt, Rinehart & Winston, 1964

11. Rieff P: The Triumph of the Therapeutic: Uses of Faith after Freud. New York, Harper Torchbooks, 1968

12. Lowe CM: Value Orientations in Counseling and Psychotherapy: The Meanings of Mental Health, second edition. Cranston, RI, Carroll Press, 1976

13. Lasch C: The Culture of Narcissism. New York, WW Norton & Co, 1978

14. Becker E: The Denial of Death. New York, Free Press, 1973

15. Kung H: Freud and the Problem of God. New Haven, CT, Yale University Press, 1979

16. Vitz PC: Psychology as Religion: The Cult of Self-Worship. Grand Rapids, MI, Erdmans, 1977

17. Durkheim E: Le Suicide Paris, 1978. Translated as, Suicide: A Study in Sociology. Translated by Spaulding JA, Simpson C. New York, Free Press, 1951

18. Harrison MH, Lazerwitz B: Do denominations matter? American Journal of Sociology 88:356–377, 1982

19. Roof WC: Socioeconomic differentials among white socioreligious groups in the United States. Social Forces 58:280–289, 1979

20. Wuthnow R: Recent patterns of secularization: a problem of generations? American Sociological Review 41:850–867, 1976

21. Hoge D: Division in the Protestant House. Philadelphia, Westminister Press, 1976

22. Etheridge FM, Feagin JR: Varieties of fundamentalism: a conceptual and empirical analysis of two Protestant denominations. Sociological Quarterly 20:37–48, 1979

23. Kaufman JH: Social correlates of spiritual maturity among North American Mennonites, in Spiritual Well-Being: Sociological Perspectives. Edited by Moberg DO. Washington, DC, University Press of America, 1979

24. Finner SL: New methods for the sociology of religion. Sociological Analysis 31:197–202, 1970

25. Himmelfarb H: Measuring religious involvement. Social Forces 53:606–618, 1975

26. Moberg DO: The development of social indicators of spiritual well-being for quality-of-life research, in Spiritual Well-Being: Sociological Perspectives. Edited by Moberg DO. Washington, DC, University Press of America, 1979

27. Hadaway CK, Roof WC: Religious commitment and the quality of life in American society. Review of Religious Research 19:295–307, 1978

28. Pattison EM: Religion and compliance, in Compliant Behavior: Beyond Obedience to Authority. Edited by Rosenbaum M. New York, Human Sciences Press, 1983

29. Roof WC: Concepts and indicators of religious commitment: a critical review, in The Religious Dimension: New Directions in Quantitative Research. Edited by Wuthnow R. New York, Academic Press, 1979

30. Gorsuch RL: The boon and bane of investigating religion. Am Psychol 39:228–236, 1984

31. Glock CY, Stark R: Religion and Society in Tension. Chicago, Rand McNally, 1965

32. Mullins CJ: A Guide to Writing and Publishing in the Social and Behavioral Sciences. New York, John Wiley & Sons, 1977

33. Warriner JE, Griffith F: English Grammar and Composition. New York, Harcourt, Brace, and World, 1965

34. Sanua VD: Religion, mental health, and personality: a review of empirical studies. Am J Psychiatry 125:1203–1213, 1969

35. Light RJ, Pillemer DB: Summing Up: The Science of Reviewing Research. Cambridge, MA, Harvard University Press, 1984

36. Buehler C, Hesser G, Weigert A: A study of articles on religion in major sociology journals. Journal for the Scientific Study of Religion 11:165–170, 1973

37. Lenski GE: The Religious Factor. Garden City, NY, Doubleday, 1961

38. Capps D, Ransohoff P, Rambo L: Publication trends in the psychology of religion to 1974. Journal for the Scientific Study of Religion 15:15–28, 1976

39. Glock CY, Bellah RN (eds): The New Religious Consciousness. Berkeley, University of California Press, 1976

40. Johnston RL: Religion in Society: A Sociology of Religion, second edition. Englewood Cliffs, NJ, Prentice-Hall, 1983

41. Remington RD, Schork MA: Statistics with Applications to the Biological and Health Sciences. Englewood Cliffs, NJ, Prentice-Hall, 1970

42. Grove WM, Andreasen NC: Simultaneous tests of many hypotheses in exploratory research. J Nerv Ment Dis 170:3–8, 1982

43. Kleinbaum DG, Kupper LL: Applied Regression Analysis and Other Multivariate Methods. North Scituate, MA, Duxbury Press, 1978

44. Shaver P, Lenauer M, Sadd S: Religiousness, conversion, and subjective well-being: the healthy-minded religion of modern American women. Am J Psychiatry 137:1563–1568, 1980

45. Hellman RE, Green R, Gray JL, et al: Childhood sexual identity, religiosity, and "homophobia" as influences in the development of transsexualism, homosexuality, and heterosexuality. Arch Gen Psychiatry 38:910–915, 1981

46. Bergin AE: Religiosity and mental health: a critical re-evaluation and meta-analysis. Professional Psychology: Research and Practice 14:170–184, 1983

47. James W: The Varieties of Religious Experience. London, Collier-Macmillan Publishers, 1961

48. Allport G: The Individual and His Religion. New York, Macmillan, 1950

49. Freud S: A religious experience, in Complete Psychological Works, Standard Edition, vol. 21. Translated and edited by Strachey J. London, Hogarth Press, 1968

50. Wallace ER: Freud and religion. Am J Psychiatry 136:237–238, 1979

51. Saltzman L: The psychology of religious and ideological conversion. Psychiatry 16:177–187, 1953

52. Bergman P: A religious conversion in the course of psychotherapy. Am J Psychother 7:41–58, 1953

53. Christensen CW: Religious conversion. Arch Gen Psychiatry 9:207–216, 1963

54. Levin TM, Zegans LS: Adolescent identity crisis and religious conversion: implications for psychotherapy. Br J Med Psychol 47:73–82, 1974

55. Vincent MO: Christianity and psychiatry: rivals or allies. Canadian Psychiatric Association Journal 20:527–532, 1975

56. Cavenar JO, Spaulding JG: Depressive disorders and religious conversions. J Nerv Ment Dis 165:209–212, 1977

57. Bragan K: The psychological gains and losses of religious conversion. Br J Med Psychol 50:177–180, 1977

58. Nicholi A: A new dimension of the youth culture. Am J Psychiatry 131:396–401, 1974

59. Wilson WP: Mental health benefits of religious salvation. Diseases of the Nervous System 33:382–386, 1972

60. Pattison EM, Pattison ML: Ex-Gays: religiously mediated change in homosexuals. Am J Psychiatry 137:1553–1562, 1980

61. Pruyser PW: Religion and psychiatry. JAMA 195:135–140, 1966

62. Hiltner S: Appraisal of religion and psychiatry since 1954. Journal of Religion and Health 4:217–227, 1965

63. Pattison EM: Psychiatry and religion circa 1978. Pastoral Psychology 27:119–141, 1978

64. Lindenthal JJ, Myers JK, Pepper MP, et al: Mental status and religious behavior. Journal for the Scientific Study of Religion 9:143–149, 1970

65. Stark R: Psychopathology and religious commitment. Review of Religious Research 12:165–176, 1971

66. Silverman W: Bibliography of measurement techniques used in the social scientific study of religion. Psychological Documents 13:7, 1983

67. Peto R, Pike NC, Armitage P, et al: Small-studies bias. British Journal of Cancer 34:585–612, 1976

68. Freiman JA: The importance of beta, the type II error, and sample size in the design and interpretation of the randomized control trial. N Engl J Med 299:690–694, 1978

69. Sacket DL: Bias in analytic research. Journal of Chronic Disease 32:51–63, 1979

70. Feinstein AR, Horowitz RI: Double standards, scientific methods, and epidemiologic research. N Engl J Med 307:1611–1617, 1982

71. Lee KL, McNeer JF, Starmer CF, et al: Clinical judgement and statistics. Circulation 61:508–515, 1980

72. Davidson JD, Knudsen DD: A new approach to religious commitment. Sociological Focus 10:151–172, 1977

73. Kuhn TS: The Structure of Scientific Revolutions. Chicago, University of Chicago Press, 1970

74. Slater E: The psychiatrist in search of science. Br J Psychiatry 122:625–636, 1973

75. Medawar PS: Advice to a Young Scientist. New York, Harper Colophon Books, 1981

76. Selltiz C, Wrightsman LS, Cook SW: Research Methods in Social Relations, third edition. New York, Holt, Rinehart & Winston, 1976